SUPER EASY LOW CARB DIET FOR BEGINNERS

1000 Days Of Healthy andSatisfying Low Carb Recipes For Any Carb-Conscious Lifestyle. 28-Day Meal Plan Included | Full Color Pictures Version

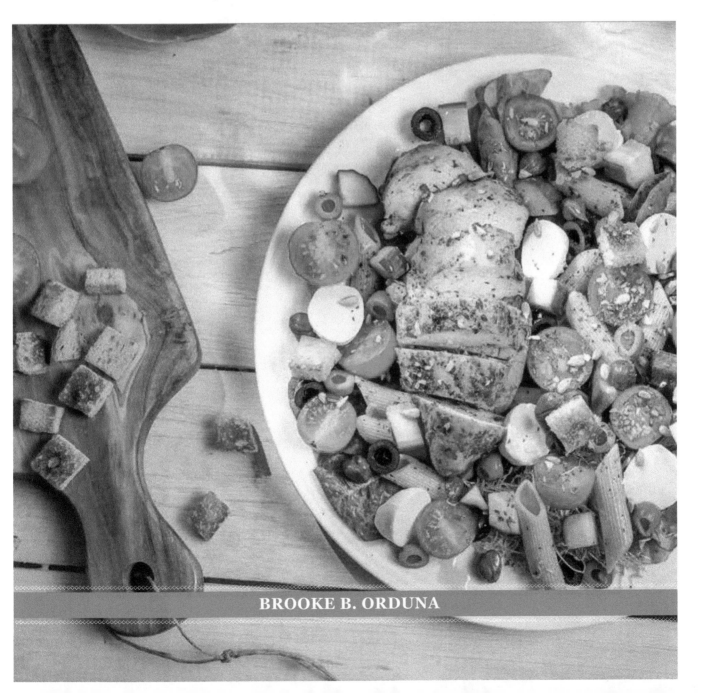

BROOKE B. ORDUNA

EDITOR: LYN

INTERIOR DESIGN: FAIZAN

COVER ART: ABR

FOOD STYLIST: JO

LOW CARBOHYDRATE DIET

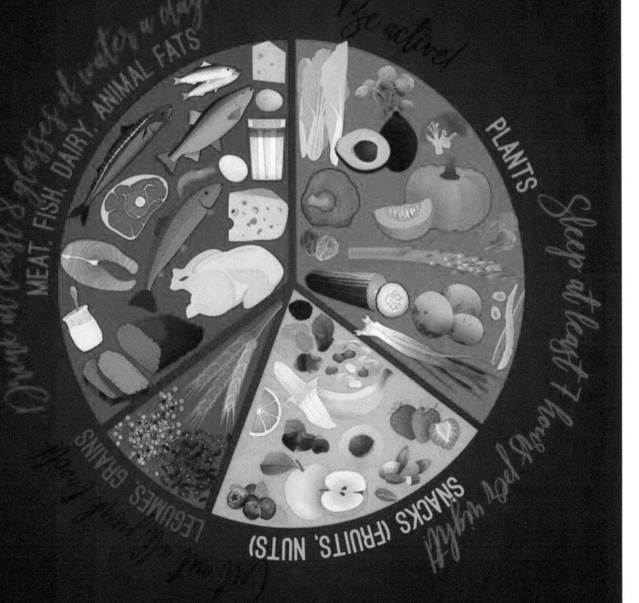

Be active!

Drink at least 8 glasses of water a day!

MEAT. FISH. DAIRY. ANIMAL FATS

PLANTS

Sleep at least 7 hours per night!

SNACKS (FRUITS, NUTS)

LEGUMES. GRAINS

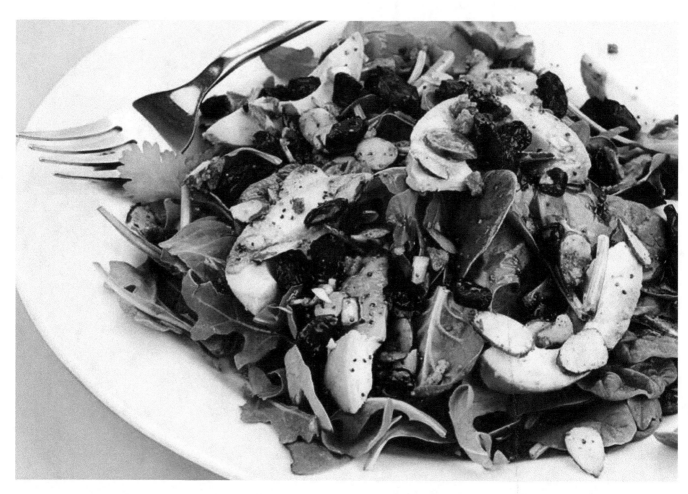

Table of Contents

Introduction   1

Chapter 1
Demystifying Low-Carb Diets   2
Understanding Carbohydrates   3
The Science Behind Low-Carb Diets   4
Potential Benefits and Risks   4

Chapter 2
Implementing a Low-Carb Diet   6
Setting Realistic Goals and Expectations   7
Transitioning to a Low-Carb Lifestyle   7
Practical Tips for Meal Planning and Grocery Shopping   7
Incorporating Exercise and Physical Activity   7

Chapter 3
28-day Meal Plan   8
Week 1   9
Week 2   10
Week 3   12
Week 4   13

Chapter 4
Breakfast   15
Bulletproof Pumpkin Spice Latte   16
Cream Cheese Pancakes   16
Raspberry Chia Smoothie   16
Blackberry-Chia Pudding   16

Berry-Avocado Smoothie   16
Coconut Chai Vanilla Smoothie   17
Cream Cheese Muffins   17
Cacao Coconut Granola   17
Kefir Strawberry Smoothie   18
Double-Pork Frittata   18
Sausage Breakfast Stacks   18
Moringa Super Green Smoothie   18
Pineapple Ginger Smoothie   19
Chocolate Hemp Smoothie   19
Bacon, Spinach, and Avocado Egg Wrap   19
Snickerdoodle Crepes   20
Smoked Salmon andCream Cheese Roll-Ups   20
Brussels Sprouts, Bacon, andEggs   20
Breakfast Quesadilla   21
Spanish Tortilla with Chorizo   21

Chapter 5
Poultry   22
Old-Fashioned Chicken Salad   23
Asian-Style Turkey Soup   23
Traditional Olla Tapada   23
Cheese and Bacon Stuffed Chicken   23
Warming Turkey and Leek Soup   24
Tangy Classic Chicken Drumettes   24
Easy Turkey Curry   24
Primavera Stuffed Turkey Fillets   25
Special Chicken Salad   25

Chicken Tikka Masala	25
Italian-Style Cocktail Meatballs	25
Spanish Spicy Chicken Salad	26
Chili Lime Chicken Bowls	26
Paprika Chicken Sandwiches	27
The Best Turkey Chili Ever	27
Oven-Baked Chicken Drumettes	27
Middle Eastern Chicken Kebabs	28
Coconut Red Curry Soup	28
Mexican Chicken Soup	28

Chapter 6
Pork, Beef & Lamb — **29**

Cream Cheese Meat Bagels	30
Sauerkraut Soup	30
Steak Fry Cups	30
Carne Asada	31
Keto Lasagna Casserole	31
Sweet-And-Sour Pork Chops	31
Balsamic Roast Beef	32
Pancetta-And-Brie–Stuffed Pork Tenderloin	32
Pork-And-Sauerkraut Casserole	32
Wild Mushroom Lamb Shanks	33
Rosemary Lamb Chops	33
Cranberry Pork Roast	33
All-In-One Lamb-Vegetable Dinner	34
Tomato-Braised Beef	34
Herb-Braised Pork Chops	34

Chapter 7
Fish & Seafood — **35**

Haddock Fillets with Mediterranean Sauce	36
Spanish Gambas al Ajillo	36
Tuna, Avocado and Ham Wraps	36
Fish Patties with Creamed Horseradish Sauce	37
Pan Fried Garlicky Fish	37
Creamy Herb Monkfish Fillets	37
Swordfish Steaks with Greek Yogurt Sauce	37
Mom's Seafood Chowder	38
Summer Salad with Cod Fish	38
Rich Fisherman's Soup	38
Traditional Fish Curry	39
Indian Chepala Vepudu	39
Stir-Fried Scallops with Vegetables	39
Cajun Shrimp Salad	40
Sea Bass with Dijon Butter Sauce	40
Creamed Monkfish Salad	40
Creole Fish Stew with Turkey Smoked Sausage	41
Salmon Salad Cups	41
Marinated and Grilled Salmon	41

Chapter 8
Sides & Snacks — **42**

Sammies With Basil Mayo	43
Keto Fat Bombs	43
Coconut Chocolate Bars	43
Keto Brownies	44
Coffee Cake	44
Keto Bread	44
Keto Chocolate Chip Cookies	45
Keto Chocolate Frosty	45
Vegan Keto Cheesecake	45

Keto Deviled Eggs	45
Keto Fudge	46
Lemon Coconut Cheesecake Fat Bombs	46
Low-Carb Burger	46
Roasted Mixed Nuts	47
Spicy Roasted Pumpkin Seeds	47
Broccoli Tabbouleh With Greek Chicken Thighs	47

Chapter 9
Vegan & Vegetarian — **48**

Cauliflower, Cheese & Collard Greens Waffles	49
Easy Chopped Salad	49
German No-Tato Salad	49
Stuffed Mushrooms	49
Speckled Salad	50
Kale Salad With Spicy Lime-Tahini Dressing	50
Oven-Roasted Asparagus with Romesco Sauce	50
Antipasto Salad	51
Spinach & Feta Frittata	51
Stuffed Mushrooms	51
Zucchini Pasta Salad	51
Tofu & Vegetable Stir-Fry	51
Roasted Cauliflower Gratin	52
Basil Spinach & Zucchini Lasagna	52
Keto Tortilla Wraps with Vegetables	52
Steamed Bok Choy with Thyme & Garlic	52
Broccoli Ginger Soup	53
Spicy Cauliflower Falafel	53
Roasted Tomatoes with Vegan Cheese Crust	53
Tofu & Hazelnut Loaded Zucchini	54
Veggie Noodles with Avocado Sauce	54
Fresh Coconut Milk Shake with Blackberries	54
Strawberry & Spinach Salad with Goat Cheese	54
Balsamic Vegetables with Feta & Almonds	55
Tasty Tofu & Swiss Chard Dip	55
Cauliflower-Based Waffles with Zucchini & Cheese	55
Tofu & Vegetable Casserole	55

Chapter 10
Desserts — **56**

Coconut Panna Cotta with Cream & Caramel	57
Superfood Red Smoothie	57
Vegan Chocolate Smoothie	57
Power Green Smoothie	57
Chocolate Mousse with Cherries	58
Strawberry Chocolate Mousse	58
Minty Lemon Tart	58
Almond Milk Berry Shake	59
No-Bake Raw Coconut Balls	59
Quick Raspberry Vanilla Shake	59
Almond Drunk Crumble	59
Peanut Butter Ice Cream	59
Refreshing Strawberry Lemonade with Basil	60
Quick Vanilla Tart	60
Cranberry Granola Bars	60
Hazelnut & Chocolate Cake	61
Grandma's Zucchini & Nut Cake	61
Sage Chocolate Cheese Cake	61

Appendix 1 Measurement Conversion Chart	**62**
Appendix 2 The Dirty Dozen and Clean Fifteen	**63**
Appendix 3 Index	**64**

Introduction

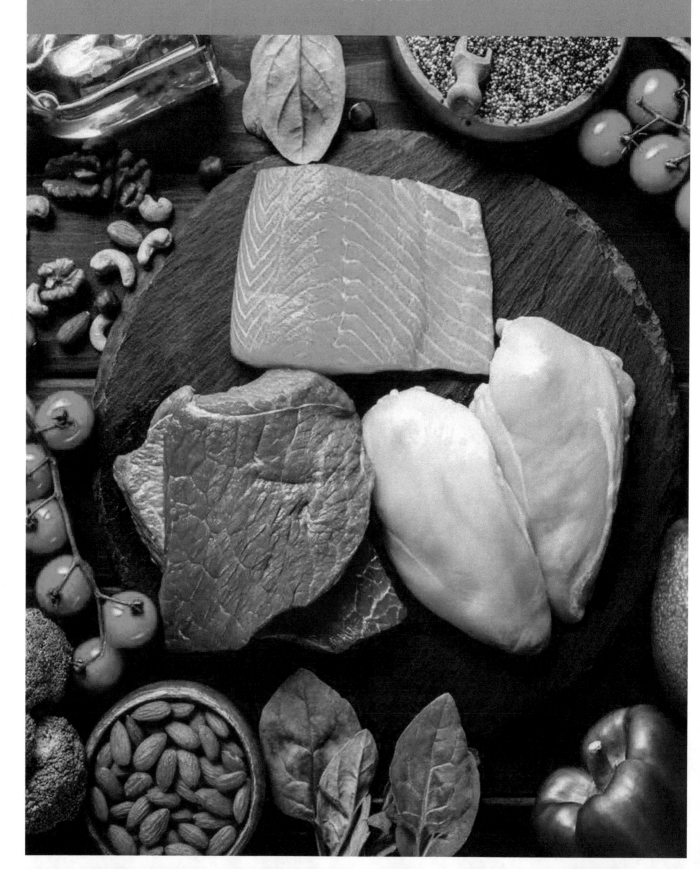

A low-carb diet is an eating plan that focuses on reducing carbohydrate intake while increasing the consumption of proteins and fats. The primary purpose of a low-carb diet is to encourage the body to burn stored fat for energy instead of relying on carbohydrates.

Low-carb diets have gained popularity in recent years. Many people are drawn to low-carb diets for various reasons, including weight loss, improved blood sugar control, and increased energy levels. Some of the popular low-carb diets, such as the ketogenic diet, have gained significant attention and have a dedicated following.

The popularity of low-carb diets can also be attributed to the increasing awareness of the potential health risks associated with excessive carbohydrate consumption, particularly refined carbohydrates and added sugars. Additionally, some studies have suggested that low-carb diets may be effective for weight loss and have positive effects on certain health markers, such as blood sugar levels and cholesterol profiles.

Typically, foods that are high in carbohydrates, such as grains, starchy vegetables, sugary foods, and some fruits, are limited or avoided in a low-carb diet. Instead, the diet emphasizes foods like meat, fish, eggs, nuts, seeds, non-starchy vegetables, and healthy fats.

The specific carbohydrate intake allowed in a low-carb diet can vary depending on the individual and the particular version of the diet. Some popular low-carb diets include the ketogenic diet (very low-carb, high-fat), Atkins diet, and the paleo diet.

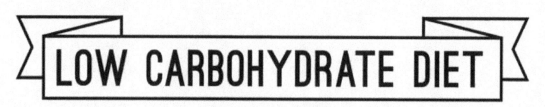

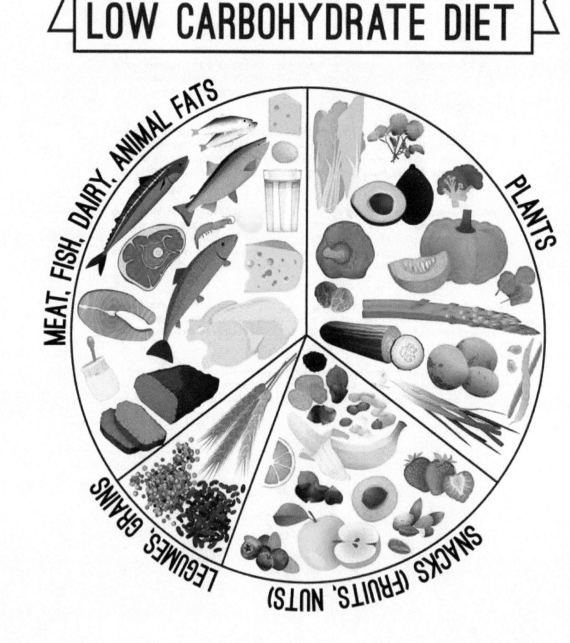

Understanding Carbohydrates

EXPLANATION OF CARBOHYDRATES AND THEIR ROLE IN THE BODY

Carbohydrates are one of the three macronutrients essential for human health, alongside proteins and fats. They serve as a vital source of energy for the body and play various other important roles.

When we consume carbohydrates through our diet, they are broken down into glucose during digestion. Glucose is then absorbed into the bloodstream and transported to cells throughout the body. It is the primary fuel source for the brain, providing the energy needed for cognitive functions and daily activities.

Carbohydrates also play a significant role in muscle function. During physical exercise, glucose stored in the muscles as glycogen is broken down and converted into energy, powering muscle contractions. Adequate carbohydrate intake is crucial for athletes and individuals engaged in regular physical activity to maintain optimal performance and prevent muscle fatigue.

Moreover, carbohydrates contribute to the regulation of blood sugar levels. When we consume carbohydrates, they raise blood sugar levels, prompting the pancreas to release insulin, a hormone that helps transport glucose from the bloodstream into cells for energy use. This process ensures that blood sugar remains within a healthy range.

Carbohydrates are not only a source of energy but also provide essential nutrients. Whole grains, fruits, and vegetables are rich in fiber, a type of carbohydrate that aids in digestion, promotes satiety, and helps maintain a healthy weight. Fiber also plays a role in reducing the risk of chronic diseases, such as heart disease and type 2 diabetes.

It's important to note that not all carbohydrates are created equal. Foods containing refined carbohydrates, such as sugary snacks and white bread, provide quick bursts of energy but lack essential nutrients and fiber. On the other hand, complex carbohydrates found in whole grains, legumes, and vegetables offer a steady release of energy, along with valuable vitamins, minerals, and fiber.

To maintain a balanced and healthy diet, it's recommended to include a variety of carbohydrates from whole food sources while considering individual needs, such as activity level and personal health goals.

DIFFERENT TYPES OF CARBOHYDRATES

Simple Carbohydrates
Simple carbohydrates are composed of one or two sugar molecules and are quickly digested and absorbed by the body, leading to a rapid rise in blood sugar levels. They are commonly found in foods such as table sugar, honey, syrups, and fruit juices. Examples of simple carbohydrates include glucose, fructose, and sucrose.

COMPLEX CARBOHYDRATES
Complex carbohydrates are composed of longer chains of sugar molecules and take longer to break down during digestion. They provide a slower and more sustained release of energy compared to simple carbohydrates. Complex carbohydrates are found in foods such as whole grains, legumes, starchy vegetables (like potatoes and corn), and whole fruits. Examples of complex carbohydrates include starch and glycogen.

DIETARY FIBER
Dietary fiber is a type of carbohydrate that cannot be fully digested by the body. Instead, it passes through the digestive system relatively intact, providing numerous health benefits. Fiber adds bulk to the diet, promotes healthy digestion, and helps regulate bowel movements. It can be found in foods such as whole grains, fruits, vegetables, nuts, and seeds. Examples of dietary fiber include cellulose, pectin, and resistant starch.

THERE ARE TWO MAIN TYPES OF DIETARY FIBER
a. Soluble Fiber
Soluble fiber dissolves in water and forms a gel-like substance in the digestive tract. It can help lower cholesterol levels, stabilize blood sugar levels, and promote a feeling of fullness. Good sources of soluble fiber include oats, barley, legumes, fruits (such as apples and citrus fruits), and vegetables (such as carrots and Brussels sprouts).

B. INSOLUBLE FIBER
Insoluble fiber does not dissolve in water and adds bulk to the stool, aiding in regular bowel movements and preventing constipation. It can be found in foods such as whole wheat, bran, nuts, seeds, and many vegetables, including broccoli, cauliflower, and green leafy vegetables.

Including a variety of carbohydrates in the diet is important for overall health. While simple carbohydrates should be consumed in moderation, complex carbohydrates and fiber-rich foods are valuable sources of nutrients and contribute to sustained energy levels, digestive health, and overall well-being.

The Science Behind Low-Carb Diets

HOW LOW-CARB DIETS WORK

Low-carb diets work by significantly reducing the intake of carbohydrates, forcing the body to shift its primary fuel source from glucose (derived from carbohydrates) to fat. By restricting carbohydrate consumption, these diets aim to promote weight loss, improve metabolic health, and provide other potential health benefits.

When carbohydrates are limited, the body's glycogen stores become depleted. Glycogen is stored glucose in the muscles and liver, which is used as a readily available energy source. As glycogen levels decrease, the body turns to alternative fuel sources to meet its energy needs.

In the absence of sufficient carbohydrates, the body starts breaking down stored fat into fatty acids and converts them into molecules called ketones through a process called ketogenesis. This metabolic state is known as ketosis. Ketones can then be used as an alternative fuel source by the brain and other organs.

IMPACT ON INSULIN LEVELS AND FAT METABOLISM

Low-carb diets can have a significant impact on insulin levels and fat metabolism. Here's how:

INSULIN LEVELS

Carbohydrate intake is the primary driver of insulin secretion in the body. When you consume carbohydrates, particularly those with a high glycemic index, they are broken down into glucose, causing blood sugar levels to rise. In response, the pancreas releases insulin to facilitate the uptake of glucose into cells for energy or storage. However, in low-carb diets, the reduced intake of carbohydrates leads to lower and more stable insulin levels.

INSULIN SENSITIVITY

Low-carb diets can improve insulin sensitivity in individuals who are overweight, obese, or have insulin resistance or type 2 diabetes. By limiting carbohydrate intake, the body requires less insulin to manage blood sugar levels. This can enhance the body's sensitivity to insulin, making it more effective in regulating blood sugar and preventing insulin resistance.

FAT METABOLISM

When carbohydrates are limited, the body turns to alternative fuel sources, such as stored fat, for energy. This is facilitated by a decrease in insulin levels. Lower insulin levels signal the body to release stored fatty acids from adipose tissue. These fatty acids are then transported to the liver, where they are converted into ketones through a process called ketogenesis. Ketones can be used as a source of energy by the brain, muscles, and other organs.

INCREASED FAT BURNING

Low-carb diets promote increased fat burning or fat oxidation. With limited carbohydrate availability, the body relies on fat stores as its primary energy source. This can lead to weight loss and a reduction in body fat.

APPETITE REGULATION

Low-carb diets are often associated with improved appetite control. Protein and fat, which are typically higher in low-carb diets, promote feelings of fullness and satisfaction, potentially reducing overall calorie intake. This can indirectly contribute to weight loss and improved fat metabolism.

Potential Benefits and Risks

BENEFITS OF A LOW-CARB DIET

WEIGHT LOSS

Low-carb diets have been shown to be effective for weight loss. By reducing carbohydrate intake, these diets can lead to decreased calorie consumption and increased fat burning, resulting in weight loss, particularly in the short term.

IMPROVED BLOOD SUGAR CONTROL

Low-carb diets can be beneficial for individuals with type 2 diabetes or insulin resistance. By limiting carbohydrate intake, they can help regulate blood sugar levels and improve insulin sensitivity.

REDUCED TRIGLYCERIDE LEVELS

Low-carb diets often lead to a decrease in blood triglyceride levels, which are associated with an increased risk of heart disease. Lowering triglyceride levels can contribute to improved cardiovascular health.

INCREASED HDL (GOOD) CHOLESTEROL

Some studies suggest that low-carb diets may raise levels of high-density lipoprotein (HDL) cholesterol, often referred to as "good" cholesterol. Higher levels of HDL cholesterol are associated with a reduced risk of heart disease.

APPETITE CONTROL

Low-carb diets can help control appetite and reduce cravings. The higher intake of protein and fat in these diets promotes feelings of satiety, which may result in reduced calorie intake.

RISKS OF A LOW-CARB DIET

NUTRITIONAL DEFICIENCIES

Severely restricting carbohydrates may lead to inadequate intake of essential nutrients, such as fiber, certain vitamins, and minerals. It's important to ensure a well-rounded, nutrient-dense diet by incorporating a variety of low-carb foods.

INCREASED FAT INTAKE

Low-carb diets often involve higher consumption of fats, including saturated fats. While some saturated fats can be part of a healthy diet, excessive intake may raise the risk of heart disease and other health problems. Choosing healthier fat sources, such as unsaturated fats, is recommended.

POTENTIAL FOR MUSCLE LOSS

Rapid weight loss associated with low-carb diets may include the loss of muscle mass. Maintaining adequate protein intake and incorporating resistance exercise can help mitigate muscle loss.

DIFFICULTY SUSTAINING LONG-TERM

Low-carb diets can be challenging to sustain over the long term due to the restrictive nature of carbohydrate intake. This may lead to difficulties with adherence and potential for weight regain if healthy eating habits are not maintained.

INDIVIDUAL VARIATIONS

People respond differently to low-carb diets, and what works well for some may not work as effectively for others. It's important to consider individual factors, such as personal health goals, preferences, and metabolic differences, when deciding on the appropriateness of a low-carb diet.

It's essential to approach any dietary change, including a low-carb diet, with caution and consult with a healthcare professional or registered dietitian to assess individual needs and potential risks. They can provide personalized guidance and help create a well-balanced eating plan that meets nutritional requirements while addressing specific health concerns.

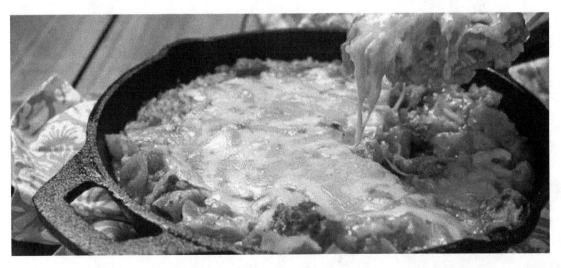

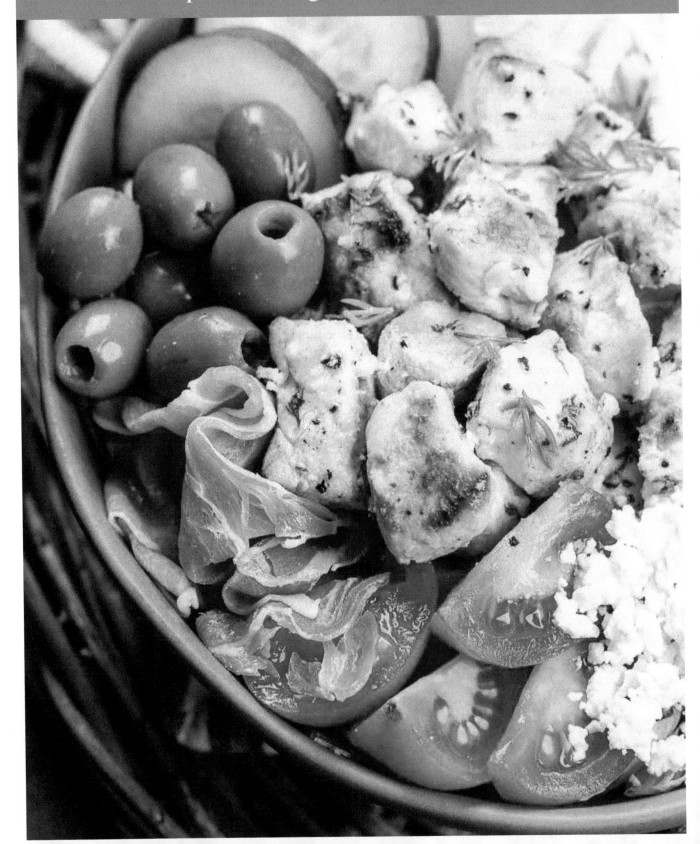

Chapter 2
Implementing a Low-Carb Diet

Setting Realistic Goals and Expectations

- Start by setting realistic goals for your low-carb diet. Determine what you hope to achieve, whether it's weight loss, better blood sugar control, or improved overall health.
- Educate yourself about the principles and guidelines of a low-carb diet to understand what to expect and how it may impact your body and lifestyle.
- Recognize that transitioning to a low-carb diet may involve some initial challenges and adjustment. Be patient with yourself and understand that it takes time to adapt to new eating habits.

Transitioning to a Low-Carb Lifestyle

- Gradually reduce your carbohydrate intake rather than making drastic changes all at once. This allows your body to adjust and helps prevent potential side effects such as fatigue or cravings.
- Identify the main sources of carbohydrates in your current diet and find low-carb alternatives. Replace processed grains and sugars with whole foods like vegetables, fruits in moderation, lean proteins, and healthy fats.
- Experiment with different low-carb recipes and meal options to find what works best for your taste preferences and dietary needs.
- Consider seeking support from a registered dietitian or joining a low-carb support group to get guidance, tips, and motivation during the transition.

Practical Tips for Meal Planning and Grocery Shopping

- Plan your meals in advance to ensure you have low-carb options readily available. This helps avoid impulsive food choices that may not align with your low-carb goals.
- Make a list of low-carb foods and ingredients you need before heading to the grocery store. Focus on fresh produce, lean meats, fish, eggs, nuts, seeds, and healthy fats like avocado and olive oil.
- Read food labels carefully to identify hidden sources of carbohydrates in packaged products. Look for added sugars, refined grains, and high-carb ingredients.
- Explore low-carb substitutes for high-carb favorites. For example, swap regular pasta with zucchini noodles (zoodles) or cauliflower rice instead of traditional rice.

Incorporating Exercise and Physical Activity

- Regular exercise is an important component of a healthy lifestyle. Incorporate both cardiovascular activities and strength training to maximize the benefits.
- Engage in activities you enjoy to make exercise more sustainable and enjoyable. This could include walking, jogging, cycling, swimming, dancing, or participating in fitness classes.
- Consult with a healthcare professional or certified fitness trainer to develop an exercise routine that suits your fitness level and health goals.
- Be mindful of your energy levels during the initial stages of transitioning to a low-carb diet. Adjust your exercise intensity and duration as needed until your body adapts to the changes.

The low-carb diet offers a promising approach to improving health and achieving weight management goals. By reducing carbohydrate intake and focusing on nutrient-dense foods, individuals can experience benefits such as enhanced weight loss, improved blood sugar control, and increased energy levels. The emphasis on whole foods and healthy fats promotes a balanced and sustainable eating pattern. While individual results may vary, adopting a low-carb diet can be a valuable tool in optimizing overall health and well-being. With its proven efficacy and delicious low-carb recipes, this dietary approach opens the door to a healthier lifestyle and a brighter future.

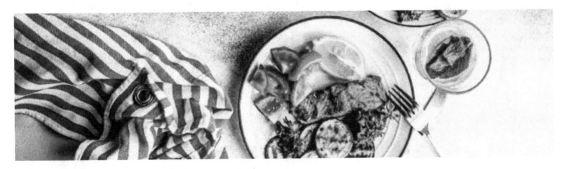

Chapter 3
28-day Meal Plan

Week 1

Congratulations on taking the first step towards a healthier you! Embarking on a low carb diet can be challenging, but remember that you have the power to transform your eating habits and improve your well-being. Embrace this week as a fresh start, where you bid farewell to processed carbs and welcome wholesome alternatives. Focus on incorporating lean proteins, leafy greens, and healthy fats into your meals. It might be tough initially, but stay determined and remind yourself of the incredible benefits you will reap from this dietary shift. Your body will thank you, and the results will soon become evident.

Meal Plan	Breakfast	Snack	Lunch	Dinner	Snack
Day-1	Raspberry Chia Smoothie	Keto Bread	Antipasto Salad	Antipasto Salad	Keto Bread
	Calories: 222 | Fat: 10g | Protein: 35g | Carbs: 8g | Fiber: 5g	Calories: 44 | Fat: 3.5g | Saturated Fat: 1.6g | Protein: 1.8g | Fiber: 0.8g	Calories: 433 | Total Fat: 38.9 g | Carbs: 13.5 g | Fiber: 4.4 g | Net Carbs: 9.1 g | Protein: 7.3 g	Calories: 433 | Total Fat: 38.9 g | Carbs: 13.5 g | Fiber: 4.4 g | Net Carbs: 9.1 g | Protein: 7.3 g	Calories: 44 | Fat: 3.5g | Saturated Fat: 1.6g | Protein: 1.8g | Fiber: 0.8g
Day-2	Raspberry Chia Smoothie	Keto Bread	Antipasto Salad	Antipasto Salad	Keto Bread
	Calories: 222 | Fat: 10g | Protein: 35g | Carbs: 8g | Fiber: 5g	Calories: 44 | Fat: 3.5g | Saturated Fat: 1.6g | Protein: 1.8g | Fiber: 0.8g	Calories: 433 | Total Fat: 38.9 g | Carbs: 13.5 g | Fiber: 4.4 g | Net Carbs: 9.1 g | Protein: 7.3 g	Calories: 433 | Total Fat: 38.9 g | Carbs: 13.5 g | Fiber: 4.4 g | Net Carbs: 9.1 g | Protein: 7.3 g	Calories: 44 | Fat: 3.5g | Saturated Fat: 1.6g | Protein: 1.8g | Fiber: 0.8g
Day-3	Cacao Coconut Granola	Keto Bread	Traditional Fish Curry	Traditional Fish Curry	Keto Bread
	Calories: 441 | Fat: 40g | Protein: 15g | Carbs: 14g | Fiber: 10g	Calories: 44 | Fat: 3.5g | Saturated Fat: 1.6g | Protein: 1.8g | Fiber: 0.8g	Calories: 209 | Fat: 6.5g | Carbs: 3.1g | Protein: 34.8g | Fiber: 0.8g	Calories: 209 | Fat: 6.5g | Carbs: 3.1g | Protein: 34.8g | Fiber: 0.8g	Calories: 44 | Fat: 3.5g | Saturated Fat: 1.6g | Protein: 1.8g | Fiber: 0.8g
Day-4	Cacao Coconut Granola	Keto Bread	Traditional Fish Curry	Traditional Fish Curry	Keto Bread
	Calories: 441 | Fat: 40g | Protein: 15g | Carbs: 14g | Fiber: 10g	Calories: 44 | Fat: 3.5g | Saturated Fat: 1.6g | Protein: 1.8g | Fiber: 0.8g	Calories: 209 | Fat: 6.5g | Carbs: 3.1g | Protein: 34.8g | Fiber: 0.8g	Calories: 209 | Fat: 6.5g | Carbs: 3.1g | Protein: 34.8g | Fiber: 0.8g	Calories: 44 | Fat: 3.5g | Saturated Fat: 1.6g | Protein: 1.8g | Fiber: 0.8g
Day-5	Cacao Coconut Granola	Keto Bread	Steak Fry Cups	Steak Fry Cups	Keto Bread

	Calories: 441 | Fat: 40g | Protein: 15g | Carbs: 14g | Fiber: 10g	Calories: 44 | Fat: 3.5g | Saturated Fat: 1.6g | Protein: 1.8g | Fiber: 0.8g	Calories: 325 | Total Fat: 19.2 g | Carbs: 12.3 g | Fiber: 6.2 g | Net Carbs: 6.1 g | Protein: 25.8 g	Calories: 325 | Total Fat: 19.2 g | Carbs: 12.3 g | Fiber: 6.2 g | Net Carbs: 6.1 g | Protein: 25.8 g	Calories: 44 | Fat: 3.5g | Saturated Fat: 1.6g | Protein: 1.8g | Fiber: 0.8g
Day-6	Sausage Breakfast Stacks	Keto Deviled Eggs	Steak Fry Cups	Steak Fry Cups	Keto Deviled Eggs
	Calories: 533 | Total Fat: 44g | Carbs: 7g | Fiber: 5g | Protein: 29g	Calories: 98 | Fat: 8.1g | Saturated Fat: 1.9g | Protein: 5.6g | Carbs: 0.5g | Fiber: 0.1g	Calories: 325 | Total Fat: 19.2 g | Carbs: 12.3 g | Fiber: 6.2 g | Net Carbs: 6.1 g | Protein: 25.8 g	Calories: 325 | Total Fat: 19.2 g | Carbs: 12.3 g | Fiber: 6.2 g | Net Carbs: 6.1 g | Protein: 25.8 g	Calories: 98 | Fat: 8.1g | Saturated Fat: 1.9g | Protein: 5.6g | Carbs: 0.5g | Fiber: 0.1g
Day-7	Sausage Breakfast Stacks	Keto Deviled Egg	Steak Fry Cups	Steak Fry Cups	Keto Deviled Eggs
	Calories: 533 | Total Fat: 44g | Carbs: 7g | Fiber: 5g | Protein: 29g	Calories: 98 | Fat: 8.1g | Saturated Fat: 1.9g | Protein: 5.6g | Carbs: 0.5g | Fiber: 0.1g	Calories: 325 | Total Fat: 19.2 g | Carbs: 12.3 g | Fiber: 6.2 g | Net Carbs: 6.1 g | Protein: 25.8 g	Calories: 325 | Total Fat: 19.2 g | Carbs: 12.3 g | Fiber: 6.2 g | Net Carbs: 6.1 g | Protein: 25.8 g	Calories: 98 | Fat: 8.1g | Saturated Fat: 1.9g | Protein: 5.6g | Carbs: 0.5g | Fiber: 0.1g

Week 2

You've made it through the first week, and now it's time to build momentum. As you continue on your low carb journey, you'll likely notice some positive changes: increased energy, improved mental clarity, and even some weight loss. This week, let's take it up a notch. Experiment with new recipes that excite your taste buds while still adhering to the low carb principles. Seek inspiration from colorful vegetables, nourishing seafood, and vibrant spices. Remember, your commitment to this healthier lifestyle is forging a path towards long-term well-being. Stay focused, and keep pushing forward!

Meal Plan	Breakfast	Snack	Lunch	Dinner	Snack
Day-1	Berry-Avocado Smoothie	Coconut Chocolate Bars	Tasty Tofu & Swiss Chard Dip	Creamed Monkfish Salad	Coconut Chocolate Bars
	Calories: 355 | Total Fat: 40g | Carbs: 16g | Fiber: 6g | Protein: 4g	Calories: 327 | Fat: 33.4g | Protein: 2.3g | Carbs: 6.2g | Fiber: 3.9g	Cal: 136 | Fat: 11g | Net Carbs: 6.3g | Protein: 3.1g	Calories: 306 | Fat: 19.4g | Carbs: 3.8g | Protein: 27g | Fiber: 0.6g	Calories: 327 | Fat: 33.4g | Protein: 2.3g | Carbs: 6.2g | Fiber: 3.9g
Day-2	Berry-Avocado Smoothie	Coconut Chocolate Bars	Tasty Tofu & Swiss Chard Dip	Creamed Monkfish Salad	Coconut Chocolate Bars

	Calories: 355 | Total Fat: 40g | Carbs: 16g | Fiber: 6g | Protein: 4g	Calories: 327 | Fat: 33.4g | Protein: 2.3g | Carbs: 6.2g | Fiber: 3.9g	Cal: 136 | Fat: 11g | Net Carbs: 6.3g | Protein: 3.1g	Calories: 306 | Fat: 19.4g | Carbs: 3.8g | Protein: 27g | Fiber: 0.6g	Calories: 327 | Fat: 33.4g | Protein: 2.3g | Carbs: 6.2g | Fiber: 3.9g
Day-3	Snickerdoodle Crepes	Coconut Chocolate Bars	Tasty Tofu & Swiss Chard Dip	Creamed Monkfish Salad	Coconut Chocolate Bars
	Calories: 434 | Fat: 42g | Protein: 12g | Carbs: 4.5g | Fiber: 1g	Calories: 327 | Fat: 33.4g | Protein: 2.3g | Carbs: 6.2g | Fiber: 3.9g	Cal: 136 | Fat: 11g | Net Carbs: 6.3g | Protein: 3.1g	Calories: 306 | Fat: 19.4g | Carbs: 3.8g | Protein: 27g | Fiber: 0.6g	Calories: 327 | Fat: 33.4g | Protein: 2.3g | Carbs: 6.2g | Fiber: 3.9g
Day-4	Snickerdoodle Crepes	Coconut Chocolate Bars	Tasty Tofu & Swiss Chard Dip	Creamed Monkfish Salad	Coconut Chocolate Bars
	Calories: 434 | Fat: 42g | Protein: 12g | Carbs: 4.5g | Fiber: 1g	Calories: 327 | Fat: 33.4g | Protein: 2.3g | Carbs: 6.2g | Fiber: 3.9g	Cal: 136 | Fat: 11g | Net Carbs: 6.3g | Protein: 3.1g	Calories: 306 | Fat: 19.4g | Carbs: 3.8g | Protein: 27g | Fiber: 0.6g	Calories: 327 | Fat: 33.4g | Protein: 2.3g | Carbs: 6.2g | Fiber: 3.9g
Day-5	Snickerdoodle Crepes	Coconut Chocolate Bars	The Best Turkey Chili Ever	Creamed Monkfish Salad	Coconut Chocolate Bars
	Calories: 434 | Fat: 42g | Protein: 12g | Carbs: 4.5g | Fiber: 1	Calories: 327 | Fat: 33.4g | Protein: 2.3g | Carbs: 6.2g | Fiber: 3.9g	Calories: 390| Fat: 25.3g | Carbs: 4.8g | Protein: 33.7g | Fiber: 1.3g	Calories: 306 | Fat: 19.4g | Carbs: 3.8g | Protein: 27g | Fiber: 0.6g	Calories: 327 | Fat: 33.4g | Protein: 2.3g | Carbs: 6.2g | Fiber: 3.9
Day-6	Snickerdoodle Crepes	Coconut Chocolate Bars	The Best Turkey Chili Ever	The Best Turkey Chili Ever	Coconut Chocolate Bars
	Calories: 434 | Fat: 42g | Protein: 12g | Carbs: 4.5g | Fiber: 1g	Calories: 327 | Fat: 33.4g | Protein: 2.3g | Carbs: 6.2g | Fiber: 3.9g	Calories: 390| Fat: 25.3g | Carbs: 4.8g | Protein: 33.7g | Fiber: 1.3g	Calories: 390| Fat: 25.3g | Carbs: 4.8g | Protein: 33.7g | Fiber: 1.3g	Calories: 327 | Fat: 33.4g | Protein: 2.3g | Carbs: 6.2g | Fiber: 3.9g
Day-7	Snickerdoodle Crepes	Almond Milk Berry Shake	The Best Turkey Chili Ever	The Best Turkey Chili Ever	Almond Milk Berry Shake
	Calories: 434 | Fat: 42g | Protein: 12g | Carbs: 4.5g | Fiber: 1g	Cal: 228g | Fat 21g | Net Carbs 5.4g | Protein 7.9g	Calories: 390| Fat: 25.3g | Carbs: 4.8g | Protein: 33.7g | Fiber: 1.3g	Calories: 390| Fat: 25.3g | Carbs: 4.8g | Protein: 33.7g | Fiber: 1.3g	Cal: 228g | Fat 21g | Net Carbs 5.4g | Protein 7.9g

Week 3

You're doing amazing! By now, you've experienced the transformative power of a low carb diet, and it's time to take things to the next level. This week, let's fine-tune your meal plan and optimize your nutrient intake. Consider incorporating more plant-based proteins like tofu or lentils, along with a variety of nuts and seeds for added crunch and healthy fats. Explore the world of low carb snacks and find options that satisfy your cravings without derailing your progress. Trust the process, stay disciplined, and remind yourself that each day brings you closer to your health goals.

Meal Plan	Breakfast	Snack	Lunch	Dinner	Snack
Day-1	Double-Pork Frittata	Vegan Keto Cheesecake	Stuffed Mushrooms	Salmon Salad Cups	Vegan Keto Cheesecake
	Calories: 437 | Total Fat: 39g | Carbs: 3g | Fiber: 0g | Protein: 21g	Calories: 328 | Fat: 29g | Protein: 8g | Carbohydrate: 11g | Fiber: 0.5g	Cal: 139 | Fat 11.2g | Net Carbs: 7.4g | Protein 4.8g	Calories: 314 | Total Fat: 26.5 gCarbs: 4.4 g | Fiber: 1.1 g | Carbs: 3.3 g | Protein: 14.6 g	Calories: 328 | Fat: 29g | Protein: 8g | Carbohydrate: 11g | Fiber: 0.5g
Day-2	Double-Pork Frittata	Vegan Keto Cheesecake	Stuffed Mushrooms	Salmon Salad Cups	Vegan Keto Cheesecake
	Calories: 437 | Total Fat: 39g | Carbs: 3g | Fiber: 0g | Protein: 21g	Calories: 328 | Fat: 29g | Protein: 8g | Carbohydrate: 11g | Fiber: 0.5g	Cal: 139 | Fat 11.2g | Net Carbs: 7.4g | Protein 4.8g	Calories: 314 | Total Fat: 26.5 gCarbs: 4.4 g | Fiber: 1.1 g | Carbs: 3.3 g | Protein: 14.6 g	Calories: 328 | Fat: 29g | Protein: 8g | Carbohydrate: 11g | Fiber: 0.5g
Day-3	Double-Pork Frittata	Vegan Keto Cheesecake	Stuffed Mushrooms	Salmon Salad Cups	Vegan Keto Cheesecake
	Calories: 437 | Total Fat: 39g | Carbs: 3g | Fiber: 0g | Protein: 21g	Calories: 328 | Fat: 29g | Protein: 8g | Carbohydrate: 11g | Fiber: 0.5g	Cal: 139 | Fat 11.2g | Net Carbs: 7.4g | Protein 4.8g	Calories: 314 | Total Fat: 26.5 gCarbs: 4.4 g | Fiber: 1.1 g | Carbs: 3.3 g | Protein: 14.6 g	Calories: 328 | Fat: 29g | Protein: 8g | Carbohydrate: 11g | Fiber: 0.5g
Day-4	Double-Pork Frittata	Vegan Keto Cheesecake	Stuffed Mushrooms	Salmon Salad Cups	Vegan Keto Cheesecake
	Calories: 437 | Total Fat: 39g | Carbs: 3g | Fiber: 0g | Protein: 21g	Calories: 328 | Fat: 29g | Protein: 8g | Carbohydrate: 11g | Fiber: 0.5g	Cal: 139 | Fat 11.2g | Net Carbs: 7.4g | Protein 4.8g	Calories: 314 | Total Fat: 26.5 gCarbs: 4.4 g | Fiber: 1.1 g | Carbs: 3.3 g | Protein: 14.6 g	Calories: 328 | Fat: 29g | Protein: 8g | Carbohydrate: 11g | Fiber: 0.5g
Day-5	Spanish Tortilla with Chorizo	Vegan Keto Cheesecake	Lemon Pork	Lemon Pork	Vegan Keto Cheesecake

Meal Plan	Breakfast	Snack	Lunch	Dinner	Snack
	Calories: 379 | Fat: 32g | Protein: 22g | Carbs: 5g | Fiber: 1g	Calories: 328 | Fat: 29g | Protein: 8g | Carbohydrate: 11g | Fiber: 0.5g	Calories: 448|Total Fat: 31g|Protein: 39g|Total Carbs: 1g|Fiber: 0g|	Calories: 448|Total Fat: 31g|Protein: 39g|Total Carbs: 1g|Fiber: 0g|	Calories: 328 | Fat: 29g | Protein: 8g | Carbohydrate: 11g | Fiber: 0.5g
Day-6	Spanish Tortilla with Chorizo	Vegan Keto Cheesecake	Lemon Pork	Lemon Pork	Vegan Keto Cheesecake
	Calories: 379 | Fat: 32g | Protein: 22g | Carbs: 5g | Fiber: 1g	Calories: 328 | Fat: 29g | Protein: 8g | Carbohydrate: 11g | Fiber: 0.5g	Calories: 448|Total Fat: 31g|Protein: 39g|Total Carbs: 1g|Fiber: 0g|	Calories: 448|Total Fat: 31g|Protein: 39g|Total Carbs: 1g|Fiber: 0g|	Calories: 328 | Fat: 29g | Protein: 8g | Carbohydrate: 11g | Fiber: 0.5g
Day-7	Spanish Tortilla with Chorizo	Quick Vanilla Tart	Lemon Pork	Lemon Pork	Quick Vanilla Tart
	Calories: 379 | Fat: 32g | Protein: 22g | Carbs: 5g | Fiber: 1g	Cal: 542 | Fat 41g | Net Carbs 8.5g | Protein 16g	Calories: 448|Total Fat: 31g|Protein: 39g|Total Carbs: 1g|Fiber: 0g|	Calories: 448|Total Fat: 31g|Protein: 39g|Total Carbs: 1g|Fiber: 0g|	Cal: 542 | Fat 41g | Net Carbs 8.5g | Protein 16g

Week 4

You've reached the final week of your low carb meal plan, and your dedication has paid off. Take a moment to reflect on how far you've come. Notice the increased vitality, improved digestion, and perhaps even a few inches shed from your waistline. As you approach the finish line, it's important to maintain your focus and continue making mindful choices. Plan your meals with intention, choosing whole foods that nourish your body and support your long-term well-being. Remember, this is not just a temporary diet but a lifestyle change. Embrace the empowerment that comes with knowing you have the ability to create lasting positive change in your life. You've got this!

Meal Plan	Breakfast	Snack	Lunch	Dinner	Snack
Day-1	Blackberry-Chia Pudding	Spicy Roasted Pumpkin Seeds	Spinach & Feta Frittata	Broccoli Ginger Soup	Spicy Roasted Pumpkin Seeds
	Calories: 437 | Total Fat: 38g | Carbs: 23g | Fiber: 15g | Protein: 8g	Calories: 246 | Fat: 22.7g | Protein: 8.5g | Carbs: 6.2g | Fiber: 1.4g	Cal: 461 | Net Carbs: 6g | Fat: 35g | Protein 26g	Calories: 344 | Fat: 26.8 g | Carbs: 12.4 g | Fiber: 4.5 g | Protein: 13.3 g	Calories: 246 | Fat: 22.7g | Protein: 8.5g | Carbs: 6.2g | Fiber: 1.4g
Day-2	Blackberry-Chia Pudding	Spicy Roasted Pumpkin Seeds	Spinach & Feta Frittata	Broccoli Ginger Soup	Spicy Roasted Pumpkin Seeds

	Calories: 437 | Total Fat: 38g | Carbs: 23g | Fiber: 15g | Protein: 8g	Calories: 246 | Fat: 22.7g | Protein: 8.5g | Carbs: 6.2g | Fiber: 1.4g	Cal: 461 | Net Carbs: 6g | Fat: 35g | Protein 26g	Calories: 344 | Fat: 26.8 g | Carbs: 12.4 g | Fiber: 4.5 g | Protein: 13.3 g	Calories: 246 | Fat: 22.7g | Protein: 8.5g | Carbs: 6.2g | Fiber: 1.4g
Day-3	Breakfast Que-sadilla	Spicy Roasted Pumpkin Seeds	Spinach & Feta Frittata	Broccoli Ginger Soup	Spicy Roasted Pumpkin Seeds
	Calories: 437 | Total Fat: 38g | Carbs: 23g | Fiber: 15g | Protein: 8g	Calories: 246 | Fat: 22.7g | Protein: 8.5g | Carbs: 6.2g | Fiber: 1.4g	Cal: 461 | Net Carbs: 6g | Fat: 35g | Protein 26g	Calories: 344 | Fat: 26.8 g | Carbs: 12.4 g | Fiber: 4.5 g | Protein: 13.3 g	Calories: 246 | Fat: 22.7g | Protein: 8.5g | Carbs: 6.2g | Fiber: 1.4g
Day-4	Breakfast Que-sadilla	Spicy Roasted Pumpkin Seeds	Spinach & Feta Frittata	Broccoli Ginger Soup	Spicy Roasted Pumpkin Seeds
	Calories: 437 | Total Fat: 38g | Carbs: 23g | Fiber: 15g | Protein: 8g	Calories: 246 | Fat: 22.7g | Protein: 8.5g | Carbs: 6.2g | Fiber: 1.4g	Cal: 461 | Net Carbs: 6g | Fat: 35g | Protein 26g	Calories: 344 | Fat: 26.8 g | Carbs: 12.4 g | Fiber: 4.5 g | Protein: 13.3 g	Calories: 246 | Fat: 22.7g | Protein: 8.5g | Carbs: 6.2g | Fiber: 1.4g
Day-5	Bacon, Spinach, and Avocado Egg Wrap	Keto Fat Bombs	Salisbury Steak	Salisbury Steak	Keto Fat Bombs
	Calories: 336 | Total Fat: 29g | Carbs: 5g | Fiber: 3g | Protein: 17g	Calories: 199 | Fat: 19g | Protein: 5.4g | Carbs: 4.1g | Fiber: 2.1g	Calories: 500|Total Fat: 39g|Protein: 33g|Total Carbs: 5g|Fiber: 2g	Calories: 500|Total Fat: 39g|Protein: 33g|Total Carbs: 5g|Fiber: 2g	Calories: 199 | Fat: 19g | Protein: 5.4g | Carbs: 4.1g | Fiber: 2.1g
Day-6	Bacon, Spinach, and Avocado Egg Wrap	Keto Fat Bombs	Salisbury Steak	Salisbury Steak	Keto Fat Bombs
	Calories: 336 | Total Fat: 29g | Carbs: 5g | Fiber: 3g | Protein: 17g	Calories: 199 | Fat: 19g | Protein: 5.4g | Carbs: 4.1g | Fiber: 2.1g	Calories: 500|Total Fat: 39g|Protein: 33g|Total Carbs: 5g|Fiber: 2g	Calories: 500|Total Fat: 39g|Protein: 33g|Total Carbs: 5g|Fiber: 2g	Calories: 199 | Fat: 19g | Protein: 5.4g | Carbs: 4.1g | Fiber: 2.1g
Day-7	Raspberry Chia Smoothie	Keto Fat Bombs	Salisbury Steak	Salisbury Steak	Keto Fat Bombs
	Calories: 222 | Fat: 10g | Protein: 35g | Carbs: 8g | Fiber: 5g	Calories: 199 | Fat: 19g | Protein: 5.4g | Carbs: 4.1g | Fiber: 2.1g	Calories: 500|Total Fat: 39g|Protein: 33g|Total Carbs: 5g|Fiber: 2g	Calories: 500|Total Fat: 39g|Protein: 33g|Total Carbs: 5g|Fiber: 2g	Calories: 199 | Fat: 19g | Protein: 5.4g | Carbs: 4.1g | Fiber: 2.1g

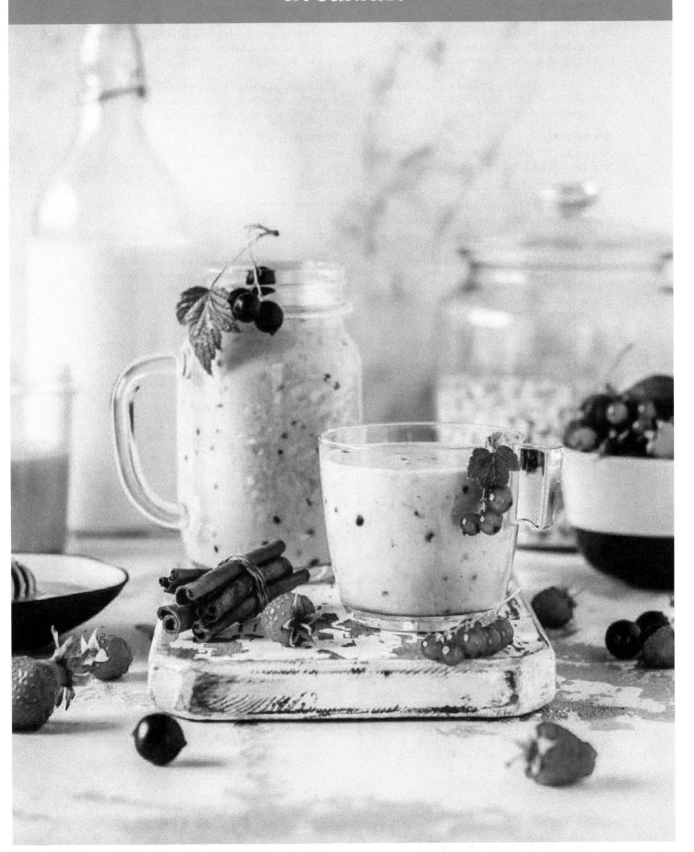

Chapter 4
Breakfast

Bulletproof Pumpkin Spice Latte

Prep time: 5 minutes | Cook time: 15 minutes | Serves 1

- 6 ounces brewed hot coffee
- 1 tablespoon coconut oil
- 1 tablespoon granulated erythritol
- 1 tablespoon solid-pack pumpkin puree
- 1 tablespoon unsalted butter
- ¼ teaspoon pumpkin pie spice

1. Place all of the ingredients in a small blender and blend until smooth. Pour into a 10-ounce mug and serve immediately.

PER SERVING

Calories: 226 | Fat: 35g | Protein:0g | Carbs: 3g | Fiber: 1g | Erythritol: 12g | Net Carbs: 2g

Cream Cheese Pancakes

Prep time: 5 minutes | Cook time: 12 minutes | Makes 4 (6-inch) pancakes

- 2 ounces cream cheese (¼ cup), softened
- 2 large eggs
- 1 teaspoon granulated erythritol
- ½ teaspoon ground cinnamon
- 1 tablespoon butter, for the pan

1. Place the cream cheese, eggs, sweetener, and cinnamon in a small blender and blend for 30 seconds, or until smooth. Let the batter rest for 2 minutes.
2. Heat the butter in a 10-inch nonstick skillet over medium heat until bubbling. Pour ¼ cup of the batter into the pan and tilt the pan in a circular motion to create a thin pancake about 6 inches in diameter. Cook for 2 minutes, or until the center is no longer glossy. Flip and cook for 1 minute on the other side. Remove and repeat with the rest of the batter, making a total of 4 pancakes.

PER SERVING

Calories: 395 | Fat: 35g | Protein: 17g | Carbs: 3g | Fiber:0g | Erythritol: 4g | Net Carbs: 3g

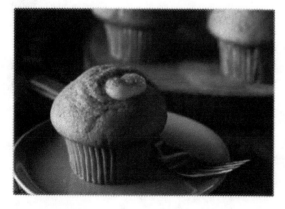

Raspberry Chia Smoothie

Prep time: 5 minutes | Cook time: 15 minutes | Serves 1

- 1 cup unsweetened vanilla-flavored almond milk
- ⅓ cup fresh raspberries
- ¼ cup sugar-free vanilla-flavored protein powder
- 2 tablespoons full-fat unsweetened coconut milk
- 1 teaspoon chia seeds
- 3 ice cubes

1. Place all of the ingredients in a blender and blend until smooth and creamy. Pour into a 12-ounce glass and serve immediately.

PER SERVING

Calories: 222 | Fat: 10g | Protein: 35g | Carbs: 8g | Fiber: 5g | Net Carbs: 3g

Blackberry-Chia Pudding

Prep time: 10 minutes | Cook time: 5 minutes | Serves 2

- 1 cup unsweetened full-fat coconut milk
- 1 teaspoon liquid stevia 1 teaspoon vanilla extract
- ½ cup blackberries, fresh or frozen (no sugar added if frozen)
- ¼ cup chia seeds

1. In a food processor (or blender), process the coconut milk, stevia, and vanilla until the mixture starts to thicken.
2. Add the blackberries, and process until thoroughly mixed and purple. Fold in the chia seeds.

PER SERVING

Calories: 437 | Total Fat: 38g | Carbs: 23g | Net Carbs: 8g | Fiber: 15g | Protein: 8g

Berry-Avocado Smoothie

Prep time: 5 minutes | Cook time: 5 minutes | Serves 2

- 1 cup unsweetened full-fat coconut milk
- 1 scoop Perfect Keto Exogenous Ketone Powder in peaches and cream
- ½ avocado
- 1 cup fresh spinach
- ½ cup berries, fresh or frozen (no sugar added if frozen)
- ½ cup ice cubes
- ¼ teaspoon liquid stevia (optional)

1. In a blender, combine the coconut milk, protein powder, avocado, spinach, berries, ice, and stevia (if using).
2. Blend until thoroughly mixed and frothy.
3. Pour into two glasses and enjoy.

PER SERVING

Calories: 355 | Total Fat: 40g | Carbs: 16g | Net Carbs: 8g | Fiber: 6g | Protein: 4g

Coconut Chai Vanilla Smoothie

Prep time: 5 minutes | Cook time: 15 minutes | Serves 1

- ½ cup brewed chai tea, cooled
- ½ cup unsweetened vanilla-flavored almond milk
- 2 tablespoons full-fat unsweetened coconut milk
- 2 tablespoons sugar-free vanilla-flavored protein powder
- 1 tablespoon granulated erythritol, or more to taste
- ¼ teaspoon pure vanilla extract
- ⅛ teaspoon ground cinnamon, plus more for garnish if desired
- 3 ice cubes

1. Place all of the ingredients in a blender and blend until smooth and creamy. Taste and add more sweetener, if desired. Pour into a 12-ounce glass and serve immediately. Garnish with a dusting of cinnamon, if desired.

PER SERVING

Calories: 170 | Fat: 8g | Protein: 18g | Carbs: 4g | Fiber: 1g | Erythritol: 12g | Net Carbs: 3g

Cream Cheese Muffins

Prep time: 10 minutes | Cook time: 10 minutes | Serves 6

- 4 tablespoons melted butter, plus more for the muffin tin
- 1 cup almond flour
- ¾ tablespoon baking powder
- 2 large eggs, lightly beaten
- 2 ounces cream cheese mixed with 2 tablespoons heavy (whipping) cream
- Handful shredded Mexican blend cheese

1. Preheat the oven to 400°F. Coat six cups of a muffin tin with butter.
2. In a small bowl, mix together the almond flour and baking powder.
3. In a medium bowl, mix together the eggs, cream cheese–heavy cream mixture, shredded cheese, and 4 tablespoons of the melted butter.
4. Pour the flour mixture into the egg mixture, and beat with a hand mixer until thoroughly mixed.
5. Pour the batter into the prepared muffin cups.
6. Bake for 12 minutes, or until golden brown on top, and serve.

PER SERVING

Calories: 247 | Total Fat: 23g | Carbs: 6g | Net Carbs: 4g | Fiber: 2g | Protein: 8g

Cacao Coconut Granola

Prep time: 5 minutes | Cook time: 30 minutes | Makes 3 cups

- ½ cup chopped raw pecans
- ½ cup flax seeds
- ½ cup superfine blanched almond flour
- ½ cup unsweetened dried coconut
- ¼ cup chopped cacao nibs
- ¼ cup chopped raw walnuts
- ¼ cup sesame seeds
- ¼ cup sugar-free vanilla-flavored protein powder
- 3 tablespoons granulated erythritol
- 1 teaspoon ground cinnamon
- ⅛ teaspoon kosher salt
- ⅓ cup coconut oil
- 1 large egg white, beaten

1. Preheat the oven to 300°F. Line a 15 by 10-inch sheet pan with parchment paper.
2. Place all of the ingredients in a large bowl. Stir well until the mixture is crumbly and holds together in small clumps. Spread out on the parchment-lined pan. Bake for 30 minutes, or until golden brown and fragrant.
3. Let the granola cool completely in the pan before removing. Store in an airtight container in the refrigerator for up to 2 weeks.

PER SERVING

Calories: 441 | Fat: 40g | Protein: 15g | Carbs: 14g | Fiber: 10g | Erythritol: 6g | Net Carbs: 4g

Kefir Strawberry Smoothie

Prep time: 5 minutes | Cook time: 15 minutes | Serves 1

- ¾ cup unsweetened vanilla-flavored almond milk
- ¼ cup full-fat unsweetened kefir, store-bought or homemade
- 1 tablespoon granulated erythritol, or more to taste
- ¼ teaspoon pure vanilla extract
- 4 medium-sized fresh strawberries, hulled (see tip), plus 1 fresh strawberry for garnish (optional)
- 3 ice cubes

1. Place all of the ingredients in a blender and blend until smooth and creamy. Taste and add more sweetener if desired. Pour into a 12-ounce glass and serve immediately. If desired, rest a strawberry on the rim for garnish.

PER SERVING

Calories: 73 | Fat: 4g | Protein: 3g | Carbs: 5g | Fiber: 1g | Erythritol: 12g | Net Carbs: 4g

Double-Pork Frittata

Prep time: 5 minutes | Cook time: 25 minutes | Serves 4

- 1 tablespoon butter or pork lard
- 8 large eggs
- 1 cup heavy (whipping) cream
- Pink Himalayan salt
- Freshly ground black pepper
- 4 ounces pancetta, chopped
- 2 ounces prosciutto, thinly sliced
- 1 tablespoon chopped fresh dill

1. Preheat the oven to 375°F. Coat a 9-by-13-inch baking pan with the butter.
2. In a large bowl, whisk the eggs and cream together. Season with pink Himalayan salt and pepper, and whisk to blend.
3. Pour the egg mixture into the prepared pan. Sprinkle the pancetta in and distribute evenly throughout.
4. Tear off pieces of the prosciutto and place on top, then sprinkle with the dill.
5. Bake for about 25 minutes, or until the edges are golden and the eggs are just set.
6. Transfer to a rack to cool for 5 minutes.
7. Cut into 4 portions and serve hot.

PER SERVING

Calories: 437 | Total Fat: 39g | Carbs: 3g | Net Carbs: 3g | Fiber: 0g | Protein: 21g

Sausage Breakfast Stacks

Prep time: 10 minutes | Cook time: 15 minutes | Serves 2

- 8 ounces ground pork
- ½ teaspoon garlic powder
- ½ teaspoon onion powder
- 2 tablespoons ghee, divided
- 2 large eggs
- 1 avocado
- Pink Himalayan salt
- Freshly ground black pepper

1. Preheat the oven to 375°F.
2. In a medium bowl, mix well to combine the ground pork, garlic powder, and onion powder. Form the mixture into 2 patties.
3. In a medium skillet over medium-high heat, melt 1 tablespoon of ghee.
4. Add the sausage patties and cook for 2 minutes on each side, until browned.
5. Transfer the sausage to a baking sheet. Cook in the oven for 8 to 10 minutes, until cooked through.
6. Add the remaining 1 tablespoon of ghee to the skillet. When it is hot, crack the eggs into the skillet and cook without disturbing for about 3 minutes, until the whites are opaque and the yolks have set.
7. Meanwhile, in a small bowl, mash the avocado.
8. Season the eggs with pink Himalayan salt and pepper.
9. Remove the cooked sausage patties from the oven.
10. Place a sausage patty on each of two warmed plates. Spread half of the mashed avocado on top of each sausage patty, and top each with a fried egg. Serve hot.

PER SERVING

Calories: 533 | Total Fat: 44g | Carbs: 7g | Net Carbs: 3g | Fiber: 5g | Protein: 29g

Moringa Super Green Smoothie

Prep time: 5 minutes | Cook time: 15 minutes | Serves 1

- 1 cup unsweetened vanilla-flavored almond milk
- 3 tablespoons full-fat unsweetened coconut milk
- 1 tablespoon pure moringa leaf powder
- 1 teaspoon granulated erythritol, or more to taste
- ¼ teaspoon pure vanilla extract
- 5 ice cubes

1. Place all of the ingredients in a blender and blend until smooth and creamy. Taste and add more sweetener if desired. Pour into a 12-ounce glass and serve immediately.

PER SERVING

Calories: 115 | Fat: 10g | Protein: 3g | Carbs: 4.5g | Fiber: 1g | Erythritol: 4g | Net Carbs: 3.5g

Pineapple Ginger Smoothie

Prep time: 8 minutes | Cook time: 15 minutes | Serves 1

- 1 cup unsweetened vanilla-flavored almond milk
- 2 tablespoons full-fat unsweetened coconut milk
- ¼ cup chopped fresh pineapple
- 2 tablespoons collagen powder
- 1 tablespoon granulated erythritol, or more to taste
- 2 teaspoons chopped fresh turmeric, or 1 teaspoon turmeric powder
- 1 teaspoon peeled and minced fresh ginger
- 3 ice cubes

1. Place all of the ingredients in a blender and blend until smooth and creamy. Taste and add more sweetener, if desired. Pour into a 12-ounce glass and serve immediately.

PER SERVING

Calories: 149 | Fat: 7g | Protein: 12g | Carbs: 9g | Fiber: 2g | Erythritol: 12g | Net Carbs: 7g

Chocolate Hemp Smoothie

Prep time: 5 minutes | Cook time: 15 minutes | Serves 1

- 1 cup unsweetened vanilla-flavored almond milk
- 2 tablespoons heavy whipping cream
- ¼ teaspoon pure vanilla extract
- ¼ cup unsweetened hemp protein powder
- 2 tablespoons unsweetened cocoa powder
- 2 tablespoons granulated erythritol, or more to taste
- 3 ice cubes

1. Place all of the ingredients in a blender and blend until smooth and creamy. Taste and add more sweetener, if desired. Pour into a 12-ounce glass and serve immediately.

PER SERVING

Calories: 245 | Fat: 17g | Protein: 15g | Carbs: 14g | Fiber: 10g | Erythritol: 24g | Net Carbs: 4g

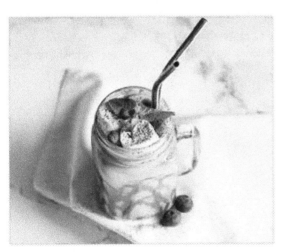

Bacon, Spinach, and Avocado Egg Wrap

Prep time: 10 minutes | Cook time: 10 minutes | Serves 2

- 6 bacon slices
- 2 large eggs
- 2 tablespoons heavy (whipping) cream
- Pink Himalayan salt
- Freshly ground black pepper
- 1 tablespoon butter, if needed
- 1 cup fresh spinach (or other greens of your choice)
- ½ avocado, sliced

1. In a medium skillet over medium-high heat, cook the bacon on both sides until crispy, about 8 minutes. Transfer the bacon to a paper towel–lined plate.
2. In a medium bowl, whisk the eggs and cream, and season with pink Himalayan salt and pepper. Whisk again to combine.
3. Add half the egg mixture to the skillet with the bacon grease.
4. Cook the egg mixture for about 1 minute, or until set, then flip with a spatula and cook the other side for 1 minute.
5. Transfer the cooked-egg mixture to a paper towel–lined plate to soak up extra grease.
6. Repeat steps 4 and 5 for the other half of the egg mixture. If the pan gets dry, add the butter.
7. Place a cooked egg mixture on each of two warmed plates. Top each with half of the spinach, bacon, and avocado slices.
8. Season with pink Himalayan salt and pepper, and roll the wraps. Serve hot.

PER SERVING

Calories: 336 | Total Fat: 29g | Carbs: 5g | Net Carbs: 2g | Fiber: 3g | Protein: 17g

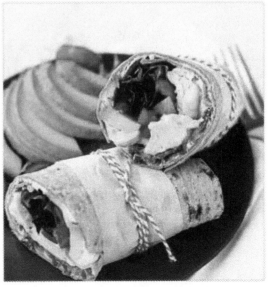

Snickerdoodle Crepes

Prep time: 8 minutes | Cook time: 24 minutes | Makes 8 crepes

FOR THE CREPES:

- 6 large eggs
- 5 ounces cream cheese (½ cup plus 1 tablespoon), softened
- 1 tablespoon granulated erythritol
- 1 teaspoon ground cinnamon
- 2 tablespoons butter, for the pan
- For the filling/topping:
- ⅓ cup granulated erythritol
- 1 tablespoon ground cinnamon
- ½ cup (1 stick) butter, softened

1. Make the crepes: Place the eggs, cream cheese, sweetener, and cinnamon in a blender and blend for 30 seconds, or until smooth. Let the batter rest for 5 minutes.
2. Heat a small pat of the butter in a 10-inch nonstick skillet over medium heat until bubbling. Pour about ¼ cup of the batter into the pan and tilt in a circular motion to create a round crepe about 6 inches in diameter. Cook for 2 minutes, or until no longer glossy in the middle. Flip and cook for 1 more minute. Remove the crepe and place on a plate or serving platter. Repeat with the remaining butter and batter to make a total of 8 crepes.
3. Meanwhile, make the filling: Mix the sweetener and cinnamon in a small bowl until combined. Place half of the cinnamon mixture and the softened butter in another small bowl. (Set the other half of the cinnamon mixture aside for the topping.) Stir with a fork until the butter is smooth and the cinnamon mixture is fully incorporated.
4. To serve, spread 1 tablespoon of the filling in the center of each crepe. Roll up each crepe and sprinkle each with 1 teaspoon of the reserved filling.

PER SERVING

Calories: 434 | Fat: 42g | Protein: 12g | Carbs: 4.5g | Fiber: 1g | Erythritol: 19g | Net Carbs: 3.5g

Smoked Salmon and Cream Cheese Roll-Ups

Prep time: 25 minutes | Cook time: 5 minutes | Serves 2

- 4 ounces cream cheese, at room temperature
- 1 teaspoon grated lemon zest
- 1 teaspoon Dijon mustard
- 2 tablespoons chopped scallions, white and green parts
- Pink Himalayan salt
- Freshly ground black pepper
- 1 (4-ounce) package cold-smoked salmon (about 12 slices)

1. Put the cream cheese, lemon zest, mustard, and scallions in a food processor (or blender), and season with pink Himalayan salt and pepper. Process until fully mixed and smooth.
2. Spread the cream-cheese mixture on each slice of smoked salmon, and roll it up. Place the rolls on a plate seam-side down.
3. Serve immediately or refrigerate, covered in plastic wrap or in a lidded container, for up to 3 days.

PER SERVING

Calories: 268 | Total Fat: 22g | Carbs: 4g | Net Carbs: 3g | Fiber: 1g | Protein: 14g

Brussels Sprouts, Bacon, and Eggs

Prep time: 5 minutes | Cook time: 20 minutes | Serves 2

- ½ pound Brussels sprouts, cleaned, trimmed, and halved
- 1 tablespoon olive oil
- Pink Himalayan salt
- Freshly ground black pepper
- Nonstick cooking spray
- 6 bacon slices, diced
- 4 large eggs
- Pinch red pepper flakes
- 2 tablespoons grated Parmesan cheese

1. Preheat the oven to 400°F.
2. In a medium bowl, toss the halved Brussels sprouts in the olive oil, and season with pink Himalayan salt and pepper.
3. Coat a 9-by-13-inch baking pan with cooking spray.
4. Put the Brussels sprouts and bacon in the pan, and roast for 12 minutes.
5. Take the pan out of the oven, and stir the Brussels sprouts and bacon. Using a spoon, create 4 wells in the mixture.
6. Carefully crack an egg into each well.
7. Season the eggs with pink Himalayan salt, black pepper, and red pepper flakes.
8. Sprinkle the Parmesan cheese over the Brussels sprouts and eggs.
9. Cook in the oven for 8 more minutes, or until the eggs are cooked to your preference, and serve.

PER SERVING

Calories: 401 | Total Fat: 29g | Carbs: 12g | Net Carbs: 7g | Fiber: 5g | Protein: 27g

Breakfast Quesadilla

Prep time: 5 minutes | Cook time: 20 minutes | Serves 2

- 2 bacon slices
- 2 large eggs
- Pink Himalayan salt
- Freshly ground black pepper
- 1 tablespoon olive oil
- 2 low-carbohydrate tortillas
- 1 cup shredded Mexican blend cheese, divided
- ½ avocado, thinly sliced

1. In a medium skillet over medium-high heat, cook the bacon on both sides until crispy, about 8 minutes. Transfer the bacon to a paper towel–lined plate to drain and cool for 5 minutes. Transfer to a cutting board, and chop the bacon.
2. Turn the heat down to medium, and crack the eggs onto the hot skillet with the bacon grease. Season with pink Himalayan salt and pepper.
3. Cook the eggs for 3 to 4 minutes, until the egg whites are set. If you want the yolks to set, you can cook them longer. Transfer the cooked eggs to a plate.
4. Pour the olive oil into the hot skillet. Place the first tortilla in the pan.
5. Add ½ cup of cheese, place slices of avocado on the cheese in a circle, top with both fried eggs, the chopped bacon, and the remaining ½ cup of cheese, and cover with the second tortilla.
6. Once the cheese starts melting and the bottom of the tortilla is golden, after about 3 minutes, flip the quesadilla. Cook for about 2 minutes on the second side, until the bottom is golden.
7. Cut the quesadilla into slices with a pizza cutter or a chef's knife and serve.

PER SERVING

Calories: 569 | Total Fat: 41g | Carbs: 27g | Net Carbs: 9g | Fiber: 18g | Protein: 27g

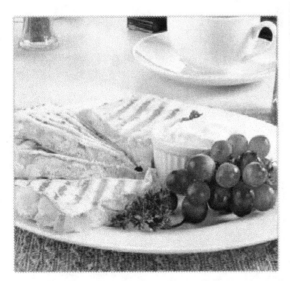

Spanish Tortilla with Chorizo

Prep time: 10 minutes | Cook time: 18 minutes | Makes 1 (10-inch) tortilla

- 8 ounces Mexican-style fresh (raw) chorizo
- 2 tablespoons avocado oil or other light-tasting oil
- 1 cup peeled and thinly sliced celery root (see notes)
- ½ cup thinly sliced yellow onions
- 1 teaspoon kosher salt
- ½ teaspoon ground black pepper
- 8 large eggs, beaten
- ½ cup shredded Manchego cheese (see notes)
- 2 tablespoons chopped fresh cilantro, for garnish (optional)

1. Remove the chorizo from the casing (if applicable) and place in a 10-inch skillet. Cook over medium heat, stirring to break into crumbles, for 5 minutes, or until cooked through. Remove the chorizo from the skillet and set aside.
2. Add the oil, celery root, and onions to the same skillet and cook over medium heat until lightly browned and softened, about 7 minutes. Season with the salt and pepper.
3. Return the cooked chorizo to the skillet and stir to combine. Reduce the heat to low. Add the beaten eggs and stir. Sprinkle with the cheese. Cook on low for 2 minutes, or until the cheese is melting.
4. Stir and bring all of the cooked egg from the sides of the skillet into the center. Stir again, then smooth the mixture back out to the edges with a rubber spatula and cook for 2 minutes, uncovered, until it's beginning to set. Cover the skillet with a lid and cook for another 2 minutes, or until the center is firm.
5. Loosen the edges with a rubber spatula and gently flip over onto a serving dish. Cut into 4 wedges and serve hot. Garnish with chopped cilantro, if desired.
6. Leftovers can be stored in an airtight container in the refrigerator for up to 5 days or in the freezer for up to 3 months. To reheat, thaw if frozen, then place in a baking dish and heat in the oven at 325°F for 8 minutes. Alternatively, you can microwave on high for 30 seconds.

PER SERVING

Calories: 379 | Fat: 32g | Protein: 22g | Carbs: 5g | Fiber: 1g | Net Carbs: 4g

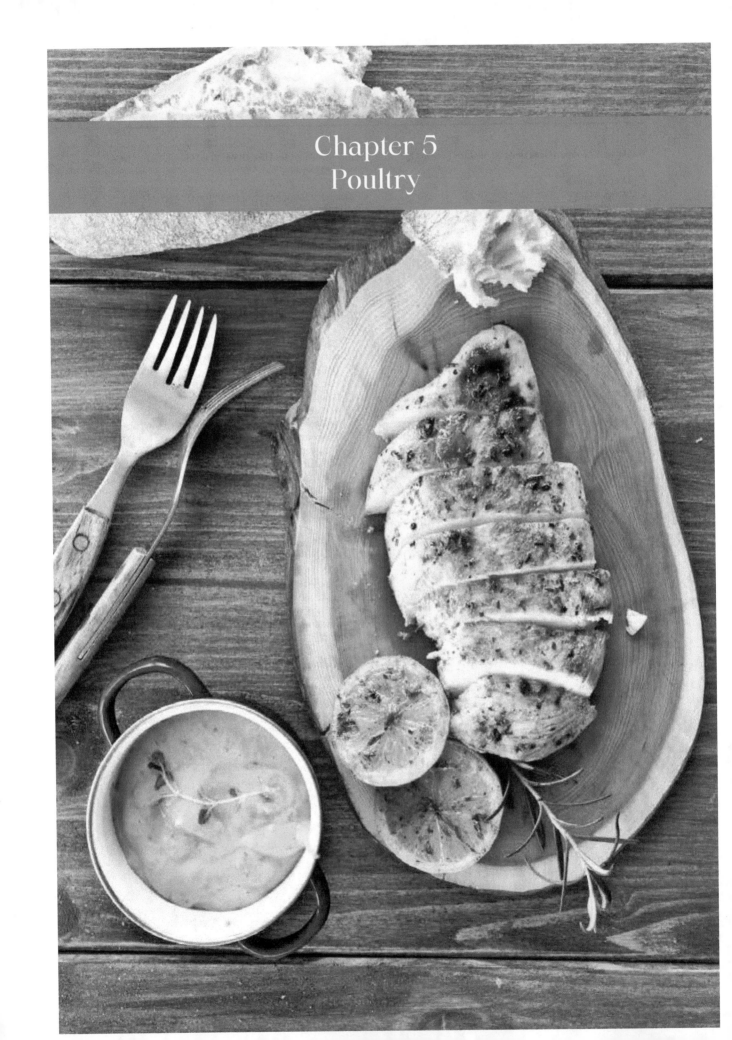

Chapter 5
Poultry

Old-Fashioned Chicken Salad

Prep time: 5 minutes | Cook time: 20 minutes |Serves 4

POACHED CHICKEN:

- 2 chicken breasts, skinless and boneless
- 1/2 teaspoon salt
- 2 bay laurels
- 1/2 teaspoon salt
- 2 bay laurels
- 1 thyme sprig
- 1 rosemary sprig
- 4 scallions, trimmed and thinly sliced
- 1 tablespoon fresh coriander, chopped
- 1 teaspoon Dijon mustard
- 2 teaspoons freshly squeezed lemon juice
- 1 cup mayonnaise, preferably homemade

1. Place all ingredients for the poached chicken in a stockpot; cover with water and bring to a rolling boil.
2. Turn the heat to medium-low and let it simmer for about 15 minutes or until a meat thermometer reads 165 degrees F. Let the poached chicken cool to room temperature.
3. Cut into strips and transfer to a nice salad bowl.
4. Toss the poached chicken with the salad ingredients; serve well chilled and enjoy!

PER SERVING

Calories: 536 | Fat: 49g | Carbs: 3.1g | Protein: 19g | Fiber: 0.5g

Asian-Style Turkey Soup

Prep time: 5 minutes | Cook time: 20 minutes |Serves 5

- 2 tablespoons canola oil
- 2 Oriental sweets peppers, deseeded and chopped
- 1 Bird's eye chili, deseeded and chopped
- 2 green onions, chopped
- 5 cups vegetable broth
- 1 pound turkey thighs, deboned and cut into halves
- 1/2 teaspoon five-spice powder
- 1 teaspoon oyster sauce
- Kosher salt, to taste

1. Heat the olive oil in a stockpot over a moderate flame. Then, sauté the peppers and onions until they have softened or about 4 minutes
2. Add in the other ingredients and bring to a boil. Turn the heat to simmer, cover, and continue to cook an additional 12 minutes.
3. Ladle into individual bowls and serve warm. Enjoy!

PER SERVING

Calories: 180 | Fat: 7.5g | Carbs: 6.7g | Protein: 21.4g | Fiber: 1.2g

Traditional Olla Tapada

Prep time: 5 minutes | Cook time: 25 minutes |Serves 3

- 2 teaspoons canola oil
- 1 red bell pepper, deveined and chopped
- 1 shallot, chopped
- 1/2 cup celery rib, chopped
- 1/2 cup chayote, peeled and cubed
- 1 pound duck breasts, boneless, skinless, and chopped into small chunks
- 1½ cups vegetable broth
- 1/2 stick Mexican cinnamon
- 1 thyme sprig
- 1 rosemary sprig
- Sea salt and freshly ground black pepper, to taste

1. Heat the canola oil in a soup pot (or clay pot) over a medium-high flame. Now, sauté the bell pepper, shallot and celery until they have softened about 5 minutes.
2. Add the remaining ingredients and stir to combine. Once it starts boiling, turn the heat to simmer and partially cover the pot.
3. Let it simmer for 17 to 20 minutes or until thoroughly cooked. Enjoy!

PER SERVING

Calories: 228 | Fat: 9.5g | Carbs: 3.3g | Protein: 30.6g | Fiber: 1g

Cheese and Bacon Stuffed Chicken

Prep time: 5 minutes | Cook time: 30 minutes |Serves 2

- 2 chicken fillets, skinless and boneless
- 1/2 teaspoon oregano
- 1/2 teaspoon tarragon
- 1/2 teaspoon paprika
- 1/4 teaspoon ground black pepper
- Sea salt, to taste
- 2 (1-ounce) slices bacon
- 2 (1-ounce) slices cheddar cheese
- 1 tomato, sliced

1. Sprinkle the chicken fillets with oregano, tarragon, paprika, black pepper, and salt.
2. Place the bacon slices and cheese on each chicken fillet. Roll up the fillets and secure with toothpicks. Place the stuffed chicken fillets on a lightly greased baking pan. Scatter the sliced tomato around the fillets.
3. Bake in the preheated oven at 390 degrees F for 15 minutes; turn on the other side and bake an additional 5 to 10 minutes or until the meat is no longer pink.
4. Discard the toothpicks and serve immediately. Bon appétit!

PER SERVING

Calories: 401 | Fat: 23.9g | Carbs: 3.7g | Protein: 41.2g | Fiber: 1.2g

Warming Turkey and Leek Soup

Prep time: 5 minutes | Cook time: 75 minutes |Serves 2

- 3 cups water
- 1/2 pound turkey thighs
- 1 cup cauliflower, broken into small florets
- 1 large-sized leek, chopped
- 1 small-sized stalk celery, chopped
- 1/2 head garlic, split horizontally
- 1/4 teaspoon turmeric powder
- 1/4 teaspoon Turkish sumac
- 1/4 teaspoon fennel seeds
- 1/2 teaspoon mustard seeds
- 1 bay laurel
- Sea salt and freshly ground black pepper, to season
- 1 teaspoon coconut aminos
- 1 whole egg

1. Add the water and turkey thighs to a pot and bring it to a rolling boil. Cook for about 40 minutes; discard the bones and shred the meat using two forks.
2. Stir in the cauliflower, leeks, celery, garlic, and spices. Reduce the heat to simmer and let it cook until everything is heated through, about 30 minutes.
3. Afterwards, add the coconut aminos and egg; whisk until the egg is well incorporated into the soup. Serve hot and enjoy!

PER SERVING

Calories: 216 | Fat: 8.1g | Carbs: 6.8g | Protein: 25.2g | Fiber: 2.1g

Tangy Classic Chicken Drumettes

Prep time: 5 minutes | Cook time: 40 minutes |Serves 4

- 1 pound chicken drumettes
- 1 tablespoon olive oil
- 2 tablespoons butter, melted
- 1 garlic cloves, sliced
- Fresh juice of 1/2 lemon
- 2 tablespoons white wine
- Salt and ground black pepper, to taste
- 1 tablespoon fresh scallions, chopped

1. Start by preheating your oven to 440 degrees F. Place the chicken in a parchment-lined baking pan. Drizzle with olive oil and melted butter.
2. Add the garlic, lemon, wine, salt, and black pepper.
3. Bake in the preheated oven for about 35 minutes. Serve garnished with fresh scallions. Enjoy!

PER SERVING

Calories: 209 | Fat: 12.2g | Carbs: 0.4g | Fiber: 0.1g | Protein: 23.2g

Easy Turkey Curry

Prep time: 5 minutes | Cook time: 1 hour |Serves 4

- 3 teaspoons sesame oil
- 1 pound turkey wings, boneless and chopped
- 2 cloves garlic, finely chopped
- 1 small-sized red chili pepper, minced
- 1/2 teaspoon turmeric powder
- 1/2 teaspoon ginger powder
- 1 teaspoon red curry paste
- 1 cup unsweetened coconut milk, preferably homemade
- 1/2 cup water
- 1/2 cup turkey consommé
- Kosher salt and ground black pepper, to taste

1. Heat sesame oil in a sauté pan. Add the turkey and cook until it is light brown about 7 minutes.
2. Add garlic, chili pepper, turmeric powder, ginger powder, and curry paste and cook for 3 minutes longer.
3. Add the milk, water, and consommé. Season with salt and black pepper. Cook for 45 minutes over medium heat. Bon appétit!

PER SERVING

Calories: 295 | Fat: 19.5g | Carbs: 2.9g | Fiber: 0g | Protein: 25.5g

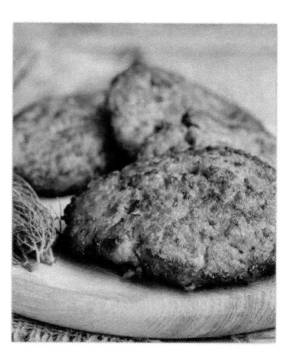

Primavera Stuffed Turkey Fillets

Prep time: 5 minutes | Cook time: 1 hour | Serves 6

- 2 tablespoons extra-virgin olive oil
- 1 tablespoon Italian seasoning mix
- Sea salt and freshly ground black pepper, to season
- 2 garlic cloves, sliced
- 6 ounces Asiago cheese, sliced
- 2 bell peppers, thinly sliced
- 1½ pounds turkey breasts
- tablespoons Italian parsley, roughly chopped

1. Brush the sides and bottom of a casserole dish with 1 tablespoon of extra-virgin olive oil. Preheat an oven to 360 degrees F.
2. Sprinkle the turkey breast with the Italian seasoning mix, salt, and black pepper on all sides.
3. Make slits in each turkey breast and stuff with garlic, cheese, and bell peppers. Drizzle the turkey breasts with the remaining tablespoon of olive oil.
4. Bake in the preheated oven for 50 minutes or until an instant-read thermometer registers 165 degrees
5. Garnish with Italian parsley and serve warm. Bon appétit!

PER SERVING

Calories: 347 | Fat: 22.2g | Carbs: 3g | Protein: 32g | Fiber: 0.5g

Special Chicken Salad

Prep time: 5 minutes | Cook time: 80 minutes | Serves 3

- 1 chicken breast, skinless
- 1/4 mayonnaise
- 1/4 cup sour cream
- 2 tablespoons Cottage cheese, room temperature
- Salt and black pepper, to taste
- 1/4 cup sunflower seeds, hulled and roasted
- 1/2 avocado, peeled and cubed
- 1/2 teaspoon fresh garlic, minced
- 2 tablespoons scallions, chopped

1. Bring a pot of well-salted water to a rolling boil.
2. Add the chicken to the boiling water; now, turn off the heat, cover, and let the chicken stand in the hot water for 15 minutes.
3. Then, drain the water; chop the chicken into bite-sized pieces. Add the remaining ingredients and mix well.
4. Place in the refrigerator for at least one hour. Serve well chilled. Enjoy!

PER SERVING

Calories: 400 | Fat: 35.1g | Carbs: 5.6g | Fiber: 2.9g | Protein: 16.1g

Chicken Tikka Masala

Prep time: 5 minutes | Cook time: 30 minutes | Serves 5

- 1½ pounds chicken breasts, cut into bite-sized pieces
- 1 onion, chopped
- 10 ounces tomato puree
- 1 teaspoon garam masala
- 1/2 cup heavy cream

1. Heat a wok that is greased with a nonstick cooking spray over medium-high heat. Now, sear the chicken breasts until golden brown on all sides.
2. Add the onions and sauté them for 2 to 3 minutes more or until tender and fragrant. Stir in the tomato puree and garam masala. Cook for 10 minutes until the sauce turns into a dark red color.
3. Fold in the heavy cream and stir to combine. Cook for 10 to 13 minutes more or until heated through.
4. Serve with cauliflower rice if desired and enjoy!

PER SERVING

Calories: 294 | Fat: 17.2g | Carbs: 4.6g | Protein: 29.3g | Fiber: 1.1g

Italian-Style Cocktail Meatballs

Prep time: 5 minutes | Cook time: 25 minutes | Serves 4

- 1 pound ground turkey
- 1 tablespoon Italian seasoning blend
- 2 cloves garlic, minced
- 1/2 cup leeks, minced
- 1 egg

1. Throw all ingredients into a mixing bowl; mix to combine well.
2. Form the mixture into bite-sized balls and arrange them on a parchment-lined baking pan. Spritz the meatballs with cooking spray.
3. Bake in the preheated oven at 395 degrees F for 18 to 22 minutes. Serve with cocktail sticks and enjoy!

PER SERVING

Calories: 216 | Fat: 11.2g | Carbs: 3.6g | Protein: 24.3g | Fiber: 0.5g

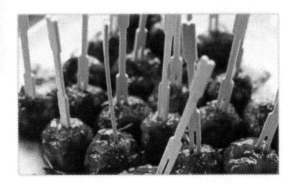

Spanish Spicy Chicken Salad

Prep time: 5 minutes | Cook time: 20 minutes |Serves 6

- 1 ½ pounds chicken breasts
- 1/2 cup dry white wine
- 1 onion, chopped
- 2 Spanish peppers, deveined and chopped
- Spanish naga chili pepper, chopped
- 2 garlic cloves, minced
- 2 cups arugula
- 1/4 cup mayonnaise
- 1 tablespoon balsamic vinegar
- 1 tablespoon stone-ground mustard
- Sea salt and freshly ground black pepper, to season

1. Place the chicken breasts in a saucepan. Add the wine to the saucepan and cover the chicken with water. Bring to a boil over medium-high heat.
2. Reduce to a simmer and cook partially covered for 10 to 14 minutes (an instant-read thermometer should register 165 degrees F).
3. Transfer the chicken from the poaching liquid to a cutting board; cut into bite-sized pieces and transfer to a salad bowl.
4. Add the remaining ingredients to the salad bowl and gently stir to combine. Serve wellchilled.

PER SERVING

Calories: 278 | Fat: 16.1g | Carbs: 4.9g | Protein: 27.2g | Fiber: 0.9g

Chili Lime Chicken Bowls

Prep time: 15 minutes | Cook time:30 minutes |Serves 4

- Cilantro Cauliflower Rice Salad:
- 1 medium head cauliflower (about 1½ lbs/680 g), or 3 cups (375 g) pre-riced cauliflower
- ⅓ packed cup (27 g) chopped fresh cilantro leaves and stems
- ¼ cup (60 ml) avocado oil
- 2 tablespoons lime juice
- 2 green onions, sliced
- ½ teaspoon finely ground sea salt
- ¼ teaspoon ground black pepper
- Chili Lime Chicken:
- 2 tablespoons avocado oil
- 1 tablespoon lime juice
- 1½ teaspoons chili powder
- 1 teaspoon garlic powder
- 2 teaspoons erythritol
- 2 teaspoons hot sauce
- ¾ teaspoon ground cumin
- ½ teaspoon paprika
- ¾ teaspoon finely ground sea salt
- ¼ teaspoon ground black pepper
- 1 pound (455 g) boneless, skinless chicken thighs

1. If you're using pre-riced cauliflower, skip ahead to Step 2. Otherwise, cut the base off the head of cauliflower and remove the florets. Transfer the florets to a food processor or blender and pulse 3 or 4 times to break them up into small (¼-inch/6-mm) pieces.
2. Put the riced cauliflower in a large saucepan and cover completely with water. Cover with the lid and bring to a boil over high heat, then reduce the heat to medium and simmer for 5 minutes, until fork-tender. (You don't want to let it get mushy!) Once done, drain, pressing the cauliflower with the back of a spoon to get out as much water as possible. Transfer the drained cauliflower to a large mixing bowl and place in the fridge to cool.
3. Make the chili lime chicken: Combine all the ingredients but the chicken thighs in a large frying pan. Whisk to combine, then add the chicken and turn to coat. Cover and set over low heat for 25 minutes, until the chicken reaches an internal temperature of 165°F (74°C).
4. After 20 minutes, pull the cooked cauliflower out of the fridge and add the remaining ingredients for the cauliflower rice salad. Toss to coat, then divide evenly among 4 bowls. Top each bowl with one-quarter of the chili lime chicken and drizzle with a bit of the pan sauce. Serve!

PER SERVING

Calories: 268 | Total Fat: 13.8 g | Saturated Fat: 2.5 g | Sodium: 454 mg | Carbs: 10.4 g | Fiber: 5 g | Net Carbs: 5.4 g | Sugars: 4 g | Protein: 25.7 g

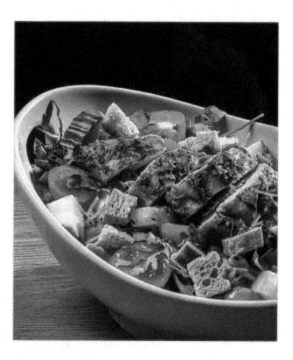

Paprika Chicken Sandwiches

Prep time: 5 minutes | Cook time:20 minutes |Serves 1

BUNS:

- 2 pounds (910 g) boneless, skinless chicken thighs
- ¼ cup (55 g) coconut oil, or ¼ cup (60 ml) avocado oil
- Sauce:
- ⅓ cup (70 g) mayonnaise
- 2 teaspoons lemon juice
- 1 clove garlic, minced
- ¾ teaspoon paprika
- ¼ teaspoon ground black pepper
- Sandwich Fillings:
- ½ cup (35 g) fresh spinach
- 8 fresh basil leaves
- 4 ounces (115 g) salami, sliced

1. Place the chicken thighs on a sheet of parchment paper. (Note: If your package of chicken thighs did not give you 8 thighs, cut the largest thigh[s] in half until you have 8 pieces.) Using a meat mallet, pound the thighs until they're ¼ inch (6 mm) thick.
2. Heat the oil in a large frying pan over medium-low heat. Add the chicken and cook for 10 minutes, then turn the chicken over and cook for another 10 minutes, or until both sides are golden and the internal temperature reaches 165°F (74°C).
3. Meanwhile, make the sauce: Place the mayonnaise, lemon juice, garlic, paprika, and pepper in a small bowl. Whisk to combine.
4. When the chicken is done, divide evenly among 4 plates, 2 pieces per plate.
5. To assemble, spread one-quarter of the sauce on one piece of chicken on each plate, then top each sauced chicken piece with one-quarter of the spinach, 2 basil leaves, and 1 ounce (28 g) of salami. Top with the second chicken piece to make sandwiches.

PER SERVING

Calories: 870 | Calories From Fat: 649 | Total Fat: 72.1 g | Saturated Fat: 35.8 g | Cholesterol: 243 mg | Sodium: 1022 mg | Carbs: 3 g | Dietary Fiber: 0.8 g | Net Carbs: 2.2 g | Sugars: 1.1 g | Protein: 52.3 g

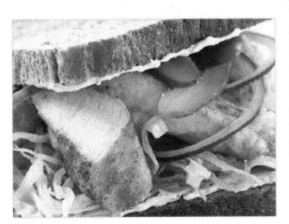

The Best Turkey Chili Ever

Prep time: 10 minutes | Cook time: 40 minutes |Serves 5

- 1 pound ground turkey 1/2 pound ground pork
- 4 tablespoons red wine
- 1 chili pepper, deveined and minced
- 2 medium Italian peppers, deveined and sliced
- 1 onion, diced
- 2 cloves garlic, minced
- 3 cups vegetable broth
- 1 vine-ripe tomato, crushed
- 1/2 teaspoon cayenne pepper
- Sea salt and ground black pepper, to your liking
- 5 ounces Monterey Jack cheese, shredded

1. Preheat a saucepan over medium-high heat. Then, brown the ground meat for 5 minutes, crumbling with a wide spatula.
2. Add in a splash of red wine to scrape up the browned bits that stick to the bottom of the saucepan.
3. Add in the remaining ingredients, except for the Monterey Jack cheese; stir to combine well. When the mixture starts to boil, turn the heat to a medium-low. Let it cook, partially covered, for 30 minutes.
4. Serve with the shredded Monterey Jack cheese. Bon appétit!

PER SERVING

Calories: 390| Fat: 25.3g | Carbs: 4.8g | Protein: 33.7g | Fiber: 1.3g

Oven-Baked Chicken Drumettes

Prep time: 5 minutes | Cook time: 40 minutes |Serves 5

- 1 tablespoon apple cider vinegar
- 1/4 cup coconut aminos
- 1 tablespoon olive oil
- 2 cloves garlic, minced
- 5 chicken drumettes
- Sea salt and ground black pepper, to taste

1. Whisk the apple cider vinegar, coconut aminos, olive oil, and garlic in a ceramic dish. Then, add the chicken drumettes to the ceramic dish and let it sit for 2 hours.
2. Discard the marinade and place the chicken drumettes in a lightly greased baking dish. Season with salt and black pepper to taste.
3. Bake in the preheated oven at 420 degrees F for 25 to 38 minutes, basting the chicken with the marinade halfway through the cooking.
4. Serve the chicken drumettes with the pan sauce and enjoy!

PER SERVING

Calories: 266 | Fat: 19.3g | Carbs: 0.8g | Protein: 20.3g | Fiber: 0.2g

Middle Eastern Chicken Kebabs

Prep time: 10 minutes | Cook time: 20 minutes | Serves 5

- 2 pounds chicken tenders, cut into bite-sized cubes
- 1/2 cup Greek-style yogurt
- 2 tablespoons coconut aminos
- 2 tablespoons extra-virgin olive oil
- 1 tablespoon mustard
- 1/2 cup tomato sauce 1/2 cup chicken stock
- 1/2 teaspoon cumin
- 1/8 teaspoon cinnamon
- 1 teaspoon salt
- 1/2 teaspoon freshly ground black pepper
- 1 teaspoon crushed red pepper flakes

1. Place all ingredients in a ceramic dish and let the chicken marinate overnight in your refrigerator.
2. Thread chicken tenders onto bamboo skewers and grill them for about 10 minutes until golden brown, turning the skewers occasionally to ensure even cooking.
3. Serve with some extra Greek yogurt if desired. Bon appétit!

PER SERVING

Calories: 274 | Fat: 10.7g | Carbs: 3.3g | Protein: 39.3g | Fiber: 0.8g

Coconut Red Curry Soup

Prep time: 10 minutes | Cook time: 20 minutes | Serves 4

- ¼ cup (55 g) coconut oil, or ¼ cup (60 ml) avocado oil
- 2 cloves garlic, minced
- 1 (2-in/5-cm) piece fresh ginger root, peeled and minced
- 2 cups (475 ml) chicken bone broth
- 1 cup (240 ml) full-fat coconut milk
- ⅓ cup (80 g) red curry paste
- 1 teaspoon finely ground sea salt
- For Serving:
- 2 medium zucchinis, spiral sliced
- 3 green onions, sliced
- ¼ cup (15 g) fresh cilantro leaves, chopped

1. Heat the oil in a large saucepan over medium-low heat. Add the garlic and ginger and cook until fragrant, about 2 minutes.
2. Add the chicken thighs, broth, coconut milk, curry paste, and salt. Stir to combine, cover, and bring to a light simmer over medium-high heat. Once simmering, reduce the heat and continue to simmer for 15 minutes, until the flavors meld.
3. Divide the spiral-sliced zucchinis among 4 bowls and top with the curry soup. Sprinkle with the green onions and cilantro before serving.

PER SERVING

Calories: 567 | Calories From Fat: 363 | Total Fat: 40.3 g | Saturated Fat: 27.2 g | Cholesterol: 101 mg | Sodium: 168 mg | Carbs: 11.3 g | Dietary Fiber: 1.5 g | Net Carbs: 9.8 g | Sugars: 3 g | Protein: 40 g

Mexican Chicken Soup

Prep time: 5 minutes | Cook time: 20 minutes | Serves 4

- ¼ cup (60 ml) avocado oil
- 1 small white onion, diced
- 2 cloves garlic, minced
- 1 red bell pepper, diced
- 1 pound (455 g) boneless, skinless chicken breasts, thinly sliced
- 1 (14½-oz/410-g) can fire-roasted whole tomatoes
- 1½ cups (355 ml) chicken bone broth
- 1 cup (240 ml) full-fat coconut milk
- 1 tablespoon apple cider vinegar
- 1 teaspoon ground cumin
- 1 teaspoon dried oregano leaves
- 1 teaspoon paprika
- ¾ teaspoon finely ground sea salt
- 1 cup (140 g) shredded cheddar cheese (dairy-free or regular) (optional)
- 2 medium Hass avocados, peeled, pitted, and sliced (about 8 oz/220 g of flesh)
- Handful of fresh cilantro leaves

1. Heat the oil in a large saucepan over medium heat. Add the onion, garlic, and bell pepper and sauté until fragrant, about 5 minutes.
2. Add the chicken, tomatoes, broth, coconut milk, vinegar, cumin, oregano, paprika, and salt. Stir to combine, cover, and bring to a light simmer over medium-high heat. Once simmering, reduce the heat and continue to simmer for 15 minutes, until the chicken is cooked through and the bell peppers are soft.
3. When the soup is done, divide evenly among 4 bowls. Top each bowl with ¼ cup (35 g) of the cheese (if using), one-quarter of the avocado slices, and a sprinkle of cilantro.

PER SERVING

Calories: 602 | Total Fat: 44.6 g | Sodium: 805 mg | Carbs: 21 g | Dietary Fiber: 13 g | Net Carbs: 8 g | Sugars: 5 g | Protein: 31.4 g

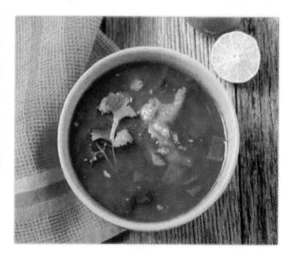

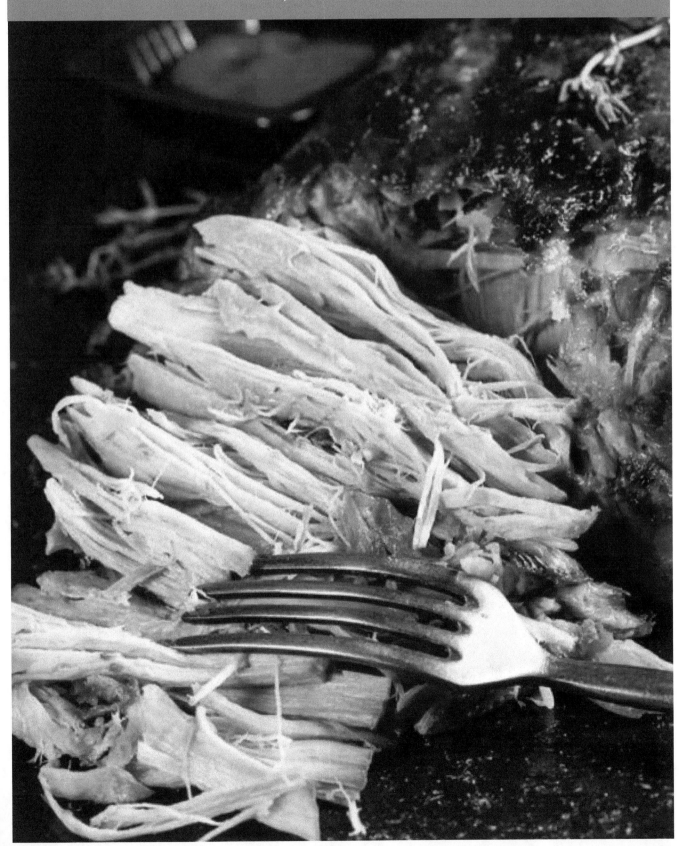

Chapter 6
Pork, Beef & Lamb

Cream Cheese Meat Bagels

Prep time: 10 minutes | Cook time:35 minutes |Serves 1

BAGELS:

- 2 tablespoons coconut oil, avocado oil, or ghee
- 2 small white onions, minced
- 2 cloves garlic, minced
- 2 pounds (910 g) ground pork
- 2 large eggs
- ½ cup (120 ml) tomato sauce
- ½ cup (35 g) nutritional yeast
- 2 teaspoons paprika
- 1½ teaspoons finely ground sea salt
- ½ teaspoon ground black pepper
- Sandwich Fillings:
- ¾ cup (6 oz/205 g) chive and onion cream cheese (dairy-free or regular)
- ½ cucumber, thinly sliced
- 6 ounces (170 g) sliced deli ham, chicken, or turkey
- 1 cup (50 g) alfalfa sprouts

1. Heat the oil in a small frying pan over medium heat. Add the onions and garlic and sauté for 10 minutes, or until fragrant.
2. Preheat the oven to 400°F (205°C). Line 2 rimmed baking sheets with parchment paper or silicone baking mats.
3. Place the ground pork, eggs, tomato sauce, nutritional yeast, paprika, salt, and pepper in a large bowl. When the onions are cooked, add them to the bowl and mix with your hands until fully incorporated.
4. Divide the meat mixture into 12 equal portions. Taking one portion at a time, roll it into a ball between your hands and press onto the lined baking sheet. Use your fingers to shape the meat mixture into a circle, keeping the thickness to about ½ inch (1.25 cm), then use your pointer finger to create a 1½-inch (4-cm) hole in the middle of the patty. Repeat with remaining meat mixture to make a total of 12 bagels, placing 6 bagels on each baking sheet.
5. Bake the bagels for 20 to 25 minutes, until the internal temperature reaches 160°F (71°C).
6. Remove from the oven and allow to cool on the pans for 30 minutes before assembling the sandwiches.
7. To assemble, spread 2 tablespoons of the cream cheese on one of the bagels. Layer on one-sixth of the cucumber slices, followed by 1 ounce (28 g) of deli meat, finishing with one-sixth of the sprouts. Top with a second bagel and repeat with remaining ingredients to make a total of 6 bagel sandwiches.

PER SERVING

Calories: 670 | Calories From Fat: 365 | Total Fat: 41 g | Saturated Fat: 14.7 g | Cholesterol: 266 mg | Sodium: 1134 mg | Carbs: 14.7 g | Dietary Fiber: 3.7 g | Net Carbs: 11 g | Sugars: 3 g | Protein: 60.7 g

Sauerkraut Soup

Prep time: 2 minutes | Cook time:25 minutes |Serves 4

- 1 pound (455 g) ground beef
- 1 small white onion, thinly sliced
- 1 clove garlic, minced
- 1¼ teaspoons ground cumin
- 3 cups (710 ml) beef bone broth
- 1 cup (235 g) sauerkraut
- ½ teaspoon finely ground sea salt

1. Place the ground beef, onion, garlic, and cumin in a saucepan. Sauté over medium heat until the onion is translucent, about 10 minutes.
2. Add the broth, sauerkraut, and salt. Cover and cook, still over medium heat, for 15 minutes, until the onion is soft and the soup is fragrant.
3. Divide the soup evenly among 4 bowls and serve.

PER SERVING

Calories: 469 | Total Fat: 27 g | Saturated Fat: 8 g | Sodium: 4150 mg | Carbs: 7.7 g | Dietary Fiber: 2.2 g | Net Carbs: 5.5 g | Sugars: 3.9 g | Protein: 48.8 g

Steak Fry Cups

Prep time: 10 minutes | Cook time:8 minutes |Serves 6

- ¼ cup plus 2 tablespoons (90 ml) avocado oil
- ¼ cup (60 ml) coconut aminos
- 2 tablespoons hot sauce
- 2 tablespoons lime juice
- 6 cloves garlic, minced
- ½ teaspoon ground black pepper
- 1 pound (455 g) top sirloin steak, cubed
- 1 red onion, diced
- 1 yellow bell pepper, sliced
- 36 endive leaves (from about 6 heads endive)
- ¼ cup (17 g) chopped fresh parsley leaves

1. Place the oil, coconut aminos, hot sauce, lime juice, garlic, and black pepper in a medium-sized bowl. Whisk to combine, then add the steak, onion, and bell pepper and toss to coat. Cover and place in the refrigerator to marinate for at least 2 hours or overnight.
2. When ready to cook the steak, transfer the entire contents of the bowl to a large frying pan. Cook over medium heat, stirring frequently, until the steak is cooked through, about 8 minutes.
3. Meanwhile, divide the endive leaves evenly among 6 plates. To serve, fill each leaf with about 2 tablespoons of the steak mixture. Sprinkle with the parsley and enjoy.

PER SERVING

Calories: 325 | Total Fat: 19.2 g | Sodium: 229 mg | Carbs: 12.3 g | Dietary Fiber: 6.2 g | Net Carbs: 6.1 g | Sugars: 2.3 g | Protein: 25.8 g

Carne Asada

Prep Time: 15 Minutes | Cook Time: 9 to 10 Hours | Serves 8

- ½ cup extra-virgin olive oil, divided
- ¼ cup lime juice
- 2 tablespoons apple cider vinegar
- 2 teaspoons minced garlic
- 1½ teaspoons paprika
- 1 teaspoon ground cumin
- 1 teaspoon chili powder
- ¼ teaspoon cayenne pepper
- 1 sweet onion cut into eighths
- 2 pounds beef rump roast
- 1 cup sour cream, for garnish

1. Lightly grease the insert of the slow cooker with 1 tablespoon of the olive oil.
2. In a small bowl, whisk together the remaining olive oil, lime juice, apple cider vinegar, garlic, paprika, cumin, chili powder, and cayenne until well blended.
3. Place the onion in the bottom of the insert and the beef on top of the vegetable. Pour the sauce over the beef.
4. Cover and cook on low for 9 to 10 hours.
5. Shred the beef with a fork.
6. Serve topped with the sour cream.

PER SERVING:

Calories: 538|Total Fat: 44g|Protein: 31g|Total Carbs: 3g|Fiber: 1g|Net Carbs: 2g|Cholesterol: 129mg

Keto Lasagna Casserole

Prep time: 10 minutes | Cook time:30 minutes |Serves 6

MEAT SAUCE:
- 3 tablespoons avocado oil, coconut oil, or ghee
- 1 pound (455 g) ground beef
- 1 (14½-oz/410-g) can fire-roasted crushed tomatoes
- 1 (6-oz/170-g) can tomato paste
- 2 teaspoons apple cider vinegar
- 2 teaspoons dried basil
- 1 teaspoon garlic powder
- 1 teaspoon dried oregano leaves
- 1 bay leaf
- ¾ teaspoon finely ground sea salt
- ½ teaspoon onion powder
- ¼ teaspoon red pepper flakes
- ¼ teaspoon dried rosemary leaves
- ¼ teaspoon dried thyme leaves
- "Cheese" Topping:
- ¼ cup (60 ml) avocado oil or melted coconut oil or ghee
- ¼ cup (60 ml) nondairy milk
- ¼ cup (17 g) nutritional yeast
- 4 large egg yolks
- 1 teaspoon Dijon mustard
- 1 teaspoon lemon juice
- ½ teaspoon garlic powder

- ½ teaspoon onion powder
- ¼ cup (10 g) fresh parsley leaves, finely chopped, for garnish

1. Heat the oil in a large frying pan over medium heat. Add the ground beef and cook until no longer pink, 5 to 7 minutes, stirring to crumble the meat as it cooks.
2. Add the crushed tomatoes, tomato paste, vinegar, basil, garlic powder, oregano, bay leaf, salt, onion powder, red pepper flakes, rosemary, and thyme. Cover and cook over low heat for 15 minutes.
3. Meanwhile, prepare the "cheese" topping: Place all the ingredients in a small bowl and whisk until smooth.
4. When the meat sauce is done, remove the bay leaf, smooth out the meat, and pour the "cheese" topping over the top.
5. Cover and cook on low for 10 minutes, or until the topping is cooked through and no longer gooey.
6. Divide among 6 plates or bowls and sprinkle with the parsley.

PER SERVING

Calories: 507 | Total Fat: 32.6 g | Sodium: 545 mg | Carbs: 18.1 g | Dietary Fiber: 5.2 g | Net Carbs: 12.9 g | Sugars: 8.3 g | Protein: 35.3 g

Sweet-And-Sour Pork Chops

Prep Time: 10 Minutes | Cook Time: 6 Hours | Serves 4

- 3 tablespoons extra-virgin olive oil, divided
- 1-pound boneless pork chops
- ½ cup granulated erythritol
- ¼ cup chicken broth
- ¼ cup tomato paste
- 2 tablespoons coconut aminos
- 2 tablespoons red chili paste
- 2 teaspoons minced garlic
- ¼ teaspoon salt
- ¼ teaspoon freshly ground black pepper

1. Lightly grease the insert of the slow cooker with 1 tablespoon of the olive oil.
2. In a large skillet over medium-high heat, heat the remaining 2 tablespoons of the olive oil. Add the pork chops, brown for about 5 minutes, and transfer to the insert.
3. In a medium bowl, stir together the erythritol, broth, tomato paste, coconut aminos, chili paste, garlic, salt, and pepper. Add the sauce to the chops.
4. Cover and cook on low for 6 hours.
5. Serve warm.

PER SERVING:

Calories: 297|Total Fat: 20g|Protein: 24g|Total Carbs: 8g|Fiber: 2g|Net Carbs: 6g|Cholesterol: 78mg

Balsamic Roast Beef

Prep Time: 15 Minutes | Cook Time: 7 to 8 Hours | Serves 8

- 3 tablespoons of extra-virgin olive oil, divided
- 2 pounds boneless beef chuck roast
- 1 cup beef broth
- ½ cup balsamic vinegar
- 1 tablespoon minced garlic
- 1 tablespoon granulated erythritol
- ½ teaspoon red pepper flakes
- 1 tablespoon chopped fresh thyme

1. Lightly grease the insert of the slow cooker with 1 tablespoon of the olive oil.
2. In a large skillet over medium-high heat, heat the remaining 2 tablespoons of the olive oil. Add the beef and brown on all sides, about 7 minutes total. Transfer to the insert.
3. In a small bowl, whisk together the broth, balsamic vinegar, garlic, erythritol, red pepper flakes, and thyme until blended.
4. Pour the sauce over the beef.
5. Cover and cook on low for 7 to 8 hours.
6. Serve warm.

PER SERVING:

Calories: 476|Total Fat: 39g|Protein: 28g|Total Carbs: 1g|Fiber: 0g|Net Carbs: 1g|Cholesterol: 117mg

Pancetta-And-Brie-Stuffed Pork Tenderloin

Prep Time: 20 Minutes | Cook Time: 8 Hours | Serves 4

- 1 tablespoon extra-virgin olive oil
- 2 (½-pound) pork tenderloins
- 4 ounces triple-cream brie
- 1 teaspoon minced garlic
- 1 teaspoon chopped fresh basil
- ⅛ teaspoon freshly ground black pepper

1. Lightly grease the insert of the slow cooker with the olive oil.
2. Place the pork on a cutting board and make a lengthwise cut, holding the knife parallel to the board, through the center of the meat without cutting right through. Open the meat up like a book and cover it with plastic wrap.
3. Pound the meat with a mallet or rolling pin until each piece is about ½ inch thick. Lay the butterflied pork on a clean work surface.
4. In a small bowl, stir together the pancetta, Brie, garlic, basil, and pepper.
5. Divide the cheese mixture between the tenderloins and spread it evenly over the meat leaving about 1 inch around the edges.
6. Roll the tenderloin up and secure with toothpicks.
7. Place the pork in the insert, cover, and cook on low for 8 hours.
8. Remove the toothpicks and serve.

PER SERVING:

Calories: 423|Total Fat: 32g|Protein: 34g|Total Carbs: 1g|Fiber: 0g|Net Carbs: 1g|Cholesterol: 132mg

Pork-And-Sauerkraut Casserole

Prep Time: 15 Minutes | Cook Time: 9 to 10 Hours | Serves 6

- 3 tablespoons extra-virgin olive oil, divided
- 2 tablespoons butter
- 2 pounds pork shoulder roast
- 1 (28-ounce) jar sauerkraut, drained
- 1 cup chicken broth
- ½ sweet onion, thinly sliced
- ¼ cup granulated erythritol

1. Lightly grease the insert of the slow cooker with 1 tablespoon of the olive oil.
2. In a large skillet over medium-high heat, heat the remaining 2 tablespoons of the olive oil and the butter. Add the pork to the skillet and brown on all sides for about 10 minutes.
3. Transfer to the insert and add the sauerkraut, broth, onion, and erythritol.
4. Cover and cook on low for 9 to 10 hours.
5. Serve warm.

PER SERVING:

Calories: 516|Total Fat: 42g|Protein: 28g|Total Carbs: 7g|Fiber: 4g|Net Carbs: 3g|Cholesterol: 117mg

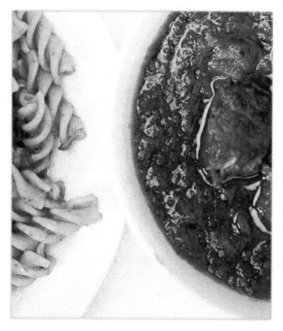

Wild Mushroom Lamb Shanks

Prep Time: 15 Minutes | Cook Time: 7 to 8 Hours | Serves 6

- 3 tablespoons extra-virgin olive oil, divided
- 2 pounds lamb shanks
- ½ pound wild mushrooms, sliced
- 1 leek, thoroughly cleaned and chopped
- 2 celery stalks, chopped
- 1 carrot, diced
- 1 tablespoon minced garlic
- 1 (15-ounce) can crushed tomatoes
- ½ cup beef broth
- 2 tablespoons apple cider vinegar
- 1 teaspoon dried rosemary
- ½ cup sour cream, for garnish

1. Lightly grease the insert of the slow cooker with 1 tablespoon of the olive oil.
2. In a large skillet over medium-high heat, heat the remaining 2 tablespoons of the olive oil. Add the lamb; brown for 6 minutes, turning once; and transfer to the insert.
3. In the skillet, sauté the mushrooms, leek, celery, carrot, and garlic for 5 minutes.
4. Transfer the vegetables to the insert along with the tomatoes, broth, apple cider vinegar, and rosemary.
5. Cover and cook on low for 7 to 8 hours.
6. Serve topped with the sour cream.

PER SERVING:

Calories: 475|Total Fat: 36g|Protein: 31g|Total Carbs: 11g|Fiber: 5g|Net Carbs: 6g|Cholesterol: 107mg

Rosemary Lamb Chops

Prep Time: 15 Minutes | Cook Time: 6 Hours | Serves 4

- 3 tablespoons extra-virgin olive oil, divided
- 1½ pounds lamb shoulder chops
- salt, for seasoning
- freshly ground black pepper, for seasoning
- ½ cup chicken broth
- 1 sweet onion, sliced
- 2 teaspoons minced garlic
- 2 teaspoons dried rosemary
- 1 teaspoon dried thyme

1. Lightly grease the insert of the slow cooker with 1 tablespoon of the olive oil.
2. In a large skillet over medium-high heat, heat the remaining 2 tablespoons of the olive oil.
3. Season the lamb with salt and pepper. Add the lamb to the skillet and brown for 6 minutes, turning once.
4. Transfer the lamb to the insert, and add the broth, onion, garlic, rosemary, and thyme.
5. Cover and cook on low for 6 hours.
6. Serve warm.

PER SERVING:

Calories: 380|Total Fat: 27g|Protein: 31g|Total Carbs: 3g|Fiber: 1g|Net Carbs: 2g|Cholesterol: 113mg

Cranberry Pork Roast

Prep Time: 15 Minutes | Cook Time: 7 to 8 Hours | Serves 6

- 3 tablespoons extra-virgin olive oil, divided
- 2 tablespoons butter
- 2 pounds pork shoulder roast
- 1 teaspoon ground cinnamon
- ¼ teaspoon allspice
- ¼ teaspoon salt
- ⅛ teaspoon freshly ground black pepper
- ½ cup cranberries
- ½ cup chicken broth
- ½ cup granulated erythritol
- 2 tablespoons dijon mustard
- juice and zest of ½ orange
- 1 scallion, white and green parts, chopped, for garnish

1. Lightly grease the insert of the slow cooker with 1 tablespoon of the olive oil.
2. In a large skillet over medium-high heat, heat the remaining 2 tablespoons of the olive oil and the butter.
3. Lightly season the pork with cinnamon, allspice, salt, and pepper. Add the pork to the skillet and brown on all sides for about 10 minutes. Transfer to the insert.
4. In a small bowl, stir together the cranberries, broth, erythritol, mustard, and orange juice and zest, and add the mixture to the pork.
5. Cover and cook on low for 7 to 8 hours.
6. Serve topped with the scallion.

PER SERVING:

Calories: 492|Total Fat: 40g|Protein: 26g|Total Carbs: 4g|Fiber: 1g|Net Carbs: 3g|Cholesterol: 117mg

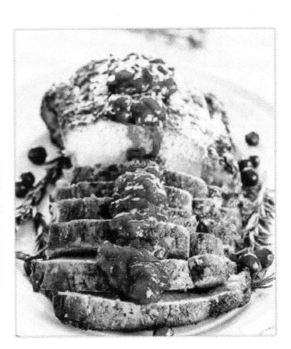

All-In-One Lamb-Vegetable Dinner

Prep Time: 10 Minutes | Cook Time: 6 Hours | Serves 4

- ¼ cup extra-virgin olive oil, divided
- 1-pound boneless lamb chops, about ½-inch thick
- salt, for seasoning
- freshly ground black pepper, for seasoning
- ½ sweet onion, sliced
- ½ fennel bulb, cut into 2-inch chunks
- 1 zucchini, cut into 1-inch chunks
- ¼ cup chicken broth
- 2 tablespoons chopped fresh basil, for garnish

1. Lightly grease the insert of the slow cooker with 1 tablespoon of the olive oil.
2. Season the lamb with salt and pepper.
3. In a medium bowl, toss together the onion, fennel, and zucchini with the remaining 3 tablespoons of the olive oil and then place half of the vegetables in the insert.
4. Place the lamb on top of the vegetables, cover with the remaining vegetables, and add the broth.
5. Cover and cook on low for 6 hours.
6. Serve topped with the basil.

PER SERVING:

Calories: 431|Total Fat: 37g|Protein: 21g|Total Carbs: 5g|Fiber: 2g|Net Carbs: 3g|Cholesterol: 80mg

Tomato-Braised Beef

Prep Time: 15 Minutes | Cook Time: 9 to 10 Hours | Serves 4

- 3 tablespoons extra-virgin olive oil, divided
- 1 pound beef chuck roast, cut into 1-inch cubes
- salt, for seasoning
- freshly ground black pepper, for seasoning
- 1 (15-ounce) can diced tomatoes
- 2 tablespoons tomato paste
- 2 teaspoons minced garlic
- 2 teaspoons dried basil
- 1 teaspoon dried oregano
- ½ teaspoon whole black peppercorns
- 1 cup shredded mozzarella cheese, for garnish
- 2 tablespoons chopped parsley, for garnish

1. Lightly grease the insert of the slow cooker with 1 tablespoon of the olive oil.
2. In a large skillet over medium-high heat, heat the remaining 2 tablespoons of the olive oil.
3. Season the beef with salt and pepper. Add the beef to the skillet and brown for 7 minutes. Transfer the beef to the insert.
4. In a medium bowl, stir together the tomatoes, tomato paste, garlic, basil, oregano, and peppercorns, and add the tomato mixture to the beef in the insert.
5. Cover and cook on low for 7 to 8 hours.
6. Serve topped with the cheese and parsley.

PER SERVING:

Calories: 539|Total Fat: 43g|Protein: 30g|Total Carbs: 7g|Fiber: 2g|Net Carbs: 5g|Cholesterol: 105mg

Herb-Braised Pork Chops

Prep Time: 15 Minutes | Cook Time: 7 to 8 Hours | Serves 6

- ¼ cup extra-virgin olive oil, divided
- 1½ pounds pork loin chops
- salt, for seasoning
- freshly ground black pepper, for seasoning
- 1 cup chicken broth
- ½ sweet onion, chopped
- 2 teaspoons minced garlic
- 1 teaspoon dried thyme
- 1 teaspoon dried oregano
- 1 cup heavy (whipping) cream
- 1 tablespoon chopped fresh basil, for garnish

1. Lightly grease the insert of the slow cooker with 1 tablespoon of the olive oil.
2. In a large skillet over medium-high heat, heat the remaining 3 tablespoons of the olive oil.
3. Lightly season the pork with salt and pepper. Add the pork to the skillet and brown for about 5 minutes. Transfer the chops to the insert.
4. In a medium bowl, stir together the broth, onion, garlic, thyme, and oregano.
5. Add the broth mixture to the chops.
6. Cover and cook on low for 7 to 8 hours.
7. Stir in the heavy cream.
8. Serve topped with the basil.

PER SERVING:

Calories: 522|Total Fat: 45g|Protein: 27g|Total Carbs: 2g|Fiber: 0g|Net Carbs: 2g|Cholesterol: 130mg

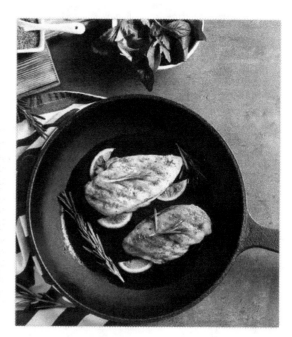

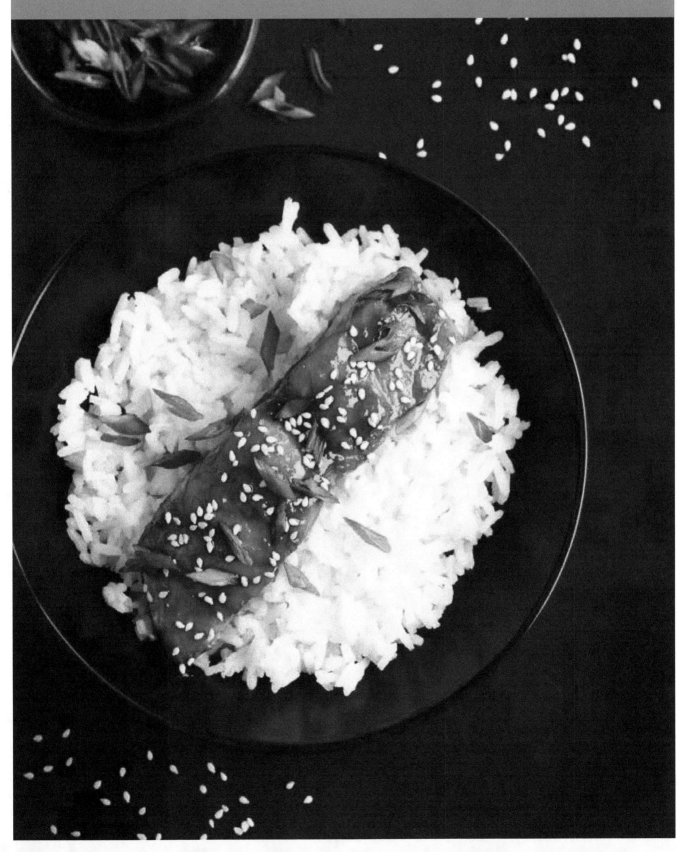

Haddock Fillets with Mediterranean Sauce

Prep time: 5 minutes | Cook time: 30 minutes |Serves 4

- 1 pound haddock fillets
- 1 tablespoon olive oil
- Sea salt and freshly cracked black pepper, to taste Mediterranean Sauce:
- 2 scallions, chopped
- 1/2 teaspoon dill weed
- 1/2 teaspoon oregano
- 1 teaspoon basil
- 1/4 cup mayonnaise
- 1/4 cup cream cheese, at room temperature

1. Start by preheating your oven to 360 degrees F. Toss the haddock fillets with the olive oil, salt, and black pepper.
2. Cover with foil and bake for 20 to 25 minutes.
3. In the meantime, make the sauce by whisking all ingredients until well combined. Serve with the warm haddock fillets and enjoy!

PER SERVING

Calories: 260 | Fat: 19.1g | Carbs: 1.3g | Protein: 19.6g | Fiber: 0.3g

Spanish Gambas al Ajillo

Prep time: 5 minutes | Cook time:15 minutes |Serves 5

- 2 tablespoons butter
- 2 cloves garlic, minced
- 2 small cayenne pepper pods
- 2 pounds shrimp, peeled and deveined
- 1/4 cup Manzanilla
- Sea salt and ground black pepper, to taste

1. Melt the butter in a sauté pan over moderate heat. Add the garlic and cayenne peppers and cook for 40 seconds.
2. Add the shrimp and cook for about a minute. Pour in the Manzanilla; season with salt and black pepper.
3. Continue to cook for a minute or so, until the shrimp are cooked through. Add lemon slices to each serving if desired. Enjoy!

PER SERVING

Calories: 203 | Fat: 5.5g | Carbs: 1.8g | Protein: 36.6g | Fiber: 0.4g

Tuna, Avocado and Ham Wraps

Prep time: 5 minutes | Cook time: 10 minutes |Serves 3

- 1/2 cup dry white wine
- 1/2 cup water
- 1/2 teaspoon mixed peppercorns
- 1/2 teaspoon dry mustard powder
- 1/2 pound ahi tuna steak
- 6 slices of ham
- 1/2 Hass avocado, peeled, pitted and sliced
- 1 tablespoon fresh lemon juice
- 6 lettuce leaves

1. Add wine, water, peppercorns, and mustard powder to a skillet and bring to a boil. Add the tuna and simmer gently for 3 minutes to 5 minutes per side.
2. Discard the cooking liquid and slice tuna into bite-sized pieces. Divide the tuna pieces between slices of ham.
3. Add avocado and drizzle with fresh lemon. Roll the wraps up and place each wrap on a lettuce leaf. Serve well chilled. Bon appétit!

PER SERVING

Calories: 308 | Fat: 19.9g | Carbs: 4.3g | Fiber: 2.5g | Protein: 27.8g

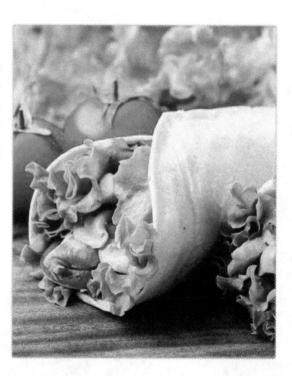

Fish Patties with Creamed Horseradish Sauce

Prep time: 5 minutes | Cook time: 20 minutes |Serves 4

- 1 pound cod fillets
- 2 eggs, beaten
- 1 tablespoon flax seeds meal
- 4 tablespoons parmesan cheese, grated
- 2 tablespoons olive oil
- 4 tablespoons mayonnaise
- 4 tablespoons Ricotta cheese
- 1 teaspoon creamed horseradish
- 2 green onions, chopped
- 1 tablespoon fresh basil, chopped

1. Steam the cod fillets until done and cooked through, approximately 10 minutes. Flake the fish with a fork; add in the beaten eggs, flax seeds meal, and parmesan.
2. Shape the mixture into 4 equal patties. Heat the olive oil in a nonstick skillet. Fry the fish patties over moderate heat for 3 minutes per side.
3. In the meantime, whisk the sauce ingredients until everything is well incorporated. Bon appétit!

PER SERVING

Calories: 346 | Fat: 23.3g | Carbs: 7g | Protein: 26.3g | Fiber: 0.7g

Pan Fried Garlicky Fish

Prep time: 5 minutes | Cook time:15 minutes |Serves 2

- 1 tablespoon olive oil
- 2 mackerel fillets
- 2 garlic cloves, minced
- Sea salt and ground black pepper, to taste
- 1/2 teaspoon thyme
- 1 teaspoon rosemary
- 1/2 teaspoon basil

1. Heat the olive oil in a frying pan over a moderate flame and swirl to coat the bottom of the pan. Pat dry the mackerel fillets.
2. Now, brown the fish fillets for 5 minutes per side until golden and crisp, shaking the pan lightly.
3. During the last minutes, add the garlic, salt, black pepper, and herbs. Bon appétit!

PER SERVING

Calories: 481 | Fat: 14.5g | Carbs: 1.1g | Protein: 80g | Fiber: 0.1g

Creamy Herb Monkfish Fillets

Prep time: 5 minutes | Cook time:20 minutes |Serves 6

- 2 tablespoons olive oil
- 6 monkfish fillets
- Sea salt and ground black pepper, to taste
- 1/2 cup sour cream
- 1 teaspoon oregano
- 1 teaspoon basil
- 1 teaspoon rosemary
- 1/2 cup cheddar cheese, shredded
- 2 tablespoons fresh chives, chopped

1. Heat the olive oil in a frying pan over a medium-high flame. Once hot, sear the monkfish fillets for 3 minutes until golden brown; flip them and cook on the other side for 3 to 4 minutes more.
2. Season with salt and black pepper. Transfer the monkfish fillets to a lightly greased casserole dish. Add the green onions and green garlic.
3. In a mixing dish, thoroughly combine the sour cream with the oregano, basil, rosemary, and cheddar cheese.
4. Spoon the mixture into your casserole dish and bake at 360 degrees F for about 11 minutes or until golden brown on top.
5. Garnish with fresh chives and serve. Bon appétit!

PER SERVING

Calories: 229 | Fat: 12.5g | Carbs: 2.2g | Protein: 25.9g | Fiber: 0.1g

Swordfish Steaks with Greek Yogurt Sauce

Prep time: 5 minutes | Cook time: 30 minutes |Serves 6

- 2 tablespoons butter
- 4 swordfish steaks
- 1 teaspoon paprika
- 1/2 teaspoon ground bay leaf
- 1 teaspoon garlic, minced
- 1 cup Greek yogurt
- 4 tablespoons mayonnaise
- 2 tablespoons fresh basil, chopped
- 2 tablespoons fresh dill, chopped
- 1 teaspoon urfa biber chile

1. Butter the bottom and sides of your casserole dish. Toss the swordfish steaks with the seasonings. Arrange the swordfish steaks in the prepared casserole dish.
2. Scatter the onion and garlic around the swordfish steaks. Bake in the preheated oven at 390 degrees F for about 25 minutes.
3. Meanwhile, whisk the Greek yogurt with the remaining ingredients to make the sauce. Serve the warm fish steaks with the sauce on the side. Bon appétit!

PER SERVING

Calories: 346 | Fat: 22.5g | Carbs: 3.2g | Protein: 31.5g | Fiber: 0.3g

Mom's Seafood Chowder

Prep time: 5 minutes | Cook time:30 minutes |Serves 4

- 2 tablespoons coconut oil
- 2 garlic cloves, pressed
- 1 shallot, chopped
- 1 cup broccoli, broken into small florets
- 2 bell peppers, chopped
- 4 cups fish broth
- 4 tablespoons dry sherry
- 6 ounces scallops
- 6 ounces shrimp, peeled and deveined
- 1 cup double cream
- 2 tablespoons fresh chives, chopped

1. Melt the coconut oil in a soup pot over a moderate flame. Now, cook the garlic and shallot for 3 to 4 minutes or until they have softened.
2. Stir in the broccoli florets, bell peppers, and fish broth; bring to a boil. Turn the heat to medium-low, partially cover, and let it cook for 12 minutes more.
3. Add in the dry sherry, scallops, shrimp, and double cream. Continue to cook an additional 7 minutes or until heated through.
4. Taste and adjust the seasonings. Serve garnished with fresh chives. Bon appétit!

PER SERVING

Calories: 272 | Fat: 19.8g | Carbs: 7g | Protein: 16.6g | Fiber: 0.7g

Summer Salad with Cod Fish

Prep time: 5 minutes | Cook time:15 minutes |Serves 5

- 4 tablespoons extra-virgin olive oil
- 5 cod fillets
- 1 tablespoon stone-ground mustard
- Sea salt and ground black pepper, to season
- 1/2 pound green cabbage, shredded
- 2 cups lettuce, cut into small pieces
- 1 red onion, sliced
- 1 garlic clove, minced
- 1 teaspoon red pepper flakes

1. Heat 1 tablespoon of the olive oil in a large frying pan over medium-high heat.
2. Once hot, fry the fish fillets for 5 minutes until golden brown; flip them and cook on the other side for 4 to 5 minutes more; work in batches to avoid overcrowding the pan.
3. Flake the cod fillets with two forks and reserve.
4. Combine the green cabbage, lettuce, onion, and garlic in a salad bowl. Dress the salad and top with the reserved fish.
5. Garnish with red pepper flakes and serve. Enjoy!

PER SERVING

Calories: 276 | Fat: 6.9g | Carbs: 6.4g | Protein: 42.7g | Fiber: 1.7g

Rich Fisherman's Soup

Prep time: 5 minutes | Cook time:25 minutes | Servin 5

- 1 tablespoons butter
- 4 scallions, chopped
- 1 cup celery, chopped
- 1 Italian pepper, deseeded and chopped
- 1 poblano pepper, deseeded and chopped
- 2 cups cauliflower, grated
- 2 Roma tomatoes, pureed
- 4 cups chicken broth
- 1 pound tilapia, skinless and chopped into small chunks
- 1/2 pound medium shrimp, deveined
- 2 tablespoons balsamic vinegar

1. Melt the butter in a heavy-bottomed pot over a moderate flame. Once hot, cook your veggies until crisp-tender or about 4 minutes, stirring periodically to ensure even cooking.
2. Add in the pureed tomatoes and chicken broth. When the soup reaches boiling, turn the heat to a simmer.
3. Add in the tilapia and let it cook, partially covered, for 12 minutes. Stir in the shrimp, partially cover, and continue to cook for 5 minutes more.
4. Afterwards, stir in the balsamic vinegar. Ladle into individual bowls and serve warm.

PER SERVING

Calories: 194 | Fat: 6.9g | Carbs: 5.6g | Protein: 26.4g | Fiber: 2.4g

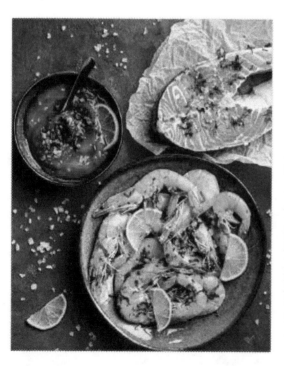

Traditional Fish Curry

Prep time: 5 minutes | Cook time:20 minutes | Servin 4

- 1 tablespoon peanut oil
- 3 green cardamoms
- 1 teaspoon cumin seeds
- 1 shallot, chopped
- 1 red chili pepper, chopped
- 1 red bell pepper, chopped
- 1 teaspoon ginger-garlic paste
- 1 cup tomato puree 1 cup chicken broth
- 1 tablespoon curry paste
- 1½ pounds tilapia
- 1 cinnamon stick
- Sea salt and ground black pepper, to taste

1. Heat the peanut oil in a saucepan over medium-heat. Now, toast the cardamoms and cumin for 2 minutes until aromatic.
2. Add in the shallot, red chili, bell pepper and continue to sauté for 2 minutes more or until just tender and translucent.
3. Add in the ginger-garlic paste and continue to sauté an additional 30 seconds. Pour the tomato puree and chicken broth into the saucepan. Bring to a boil.
4. Turn the heat to medium-low and stir in the curry paste, tilapia, cinnamon, salt, and black pepper. Let it simmer, partially covered, for 10 minutes more.
5. Flake the fish and serve in individual bowls. Enjoy!

PER SERVING

Calories: 209 | Fat: 6.5g | Carbs: 3.1g | Protein: 34.8g | Fiber: 0.8g

Indian Chepala Vepudu

Prep time: 5 minutes | Cook time:15 minutes | Servin 3

- 3 carp fillets
- 1 teaspoon chili powder
- 1 teaspoon cumin powder
- 1 teaspoon turmeric powder
- 1 coriander powder
- 1/2 teaspoon garam masala
- 1/2 teaspoon flaky salt
- 1/4 teaspoon cayenne pepper
- 3 tablespoons full-fat coconut milk
- 1 egg
- 2 tablespoons olive oil
- 6 curry leaves, for garnish

1. Pat the fish fillets with kitchen towels and add to a large resealable bag. Add the spices to the bag and shake to coat on all sides.
2. In a shallow dish, whisk the coconut milk and egg until frothy and well combined. Dip the fillets into the egg mixture.
3. Then, heat the oil in a large frying pan. Fry the

fish fillets on both sides until they are cooked through and the coating becomes crispy.
4. Serve with curry leaves and enjoy!

PER SERVING

Calories: 443 | Fat: 28.3g | Carbs: 2.6g | Protein: 42.5g | Fiber: 1g

Stir-Fried Scallops with Vegetables

Prep time: 5 minutes | Cook time: 15 minutes |Serves 5

- 1 tablespoon butter
- 2 medium Italian peppers, deveined and sliced
- 2 cups cauliflower florets
- 1/2 teaspoon fresh ginger, minced
- 1 teaspoon garlic, minced
- 2 pounds sea scallops
- 1/2 cup dry white wine
- 1/2 teaspoon cayenne pepper
- 1/2 teaspoon oregano
- 1/2 teaspoon marjoram
- 1/2 teaspoon rosemary
- Sea salt and ground black pepper, to taste
- 1/2 cup chicken broth

1. Melt the butter in a large frying pan over medium-high heat.
2. Stir in the Italian peppers, cauliflower, ginger, and garlic. Cook for about 3 minutes or until the vegetables have softened.
3. Stir in the sea scallops and continue to cook for 3 minutes. Stir to coat with the vegetable mixture.
4. Add in the remaining ingredients and let it simmer, partially covered, for a few minutes longer. Bon appétit!

PER SERVING

Calories: 217 | Fat: 3.5g | Carbs: 4.8g | Protein: 23.5g | Fiber: 1.2g

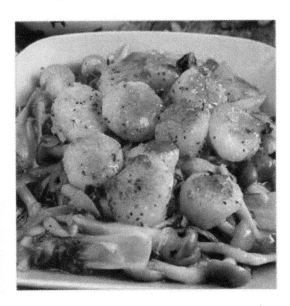

Cajun Shrimp Salad

Prep time: 5 minutes | Cook time:15 minutes |Serves 4

- 1 pound (455 g) large shrimp, peeled and deveined
- 2 tablespoons avocado oil
- 2 cloves garlic, minced
- 2 teaspoons dried basil
- 1 teaspoon dried thyme leaves
- 1¾ teaspoons paprika
- ¾ teaspoon ground black pepper
- ½ teaspoon finely ground sea salt
- ⅛ teaspoon cayenne pepper
- 1 bunch asparagus, woody ends snapped off, cut in half crosswise
- Salad:
- 1 large head butter lettuce, chopped
- 1 medium Hass avocado, peeled, pitted, and sliced (about 4 oz/110 g of flesh)
- 1 small red onion, thinly sliced
- ½ cup (120 ml) creamy Italian dressing or other creamy salad dressing of choice

1. Place the shrimp, oil, garlic, basil, thyme, paprika, black pepper, salt, and cayenne in a large frying pan. Toss to coat the shrimp, then turn the heat to medium and cook until the shrimp is pink, about 5 minutes.
2. Add the asparagus, cover, and cook for 10 minutes, or until the asparagus is fork-tender.
3. Meanwhile, divide the lettuce, avocado, and onion evenly among 4 salad plates. When the shrimp and asparagus are done, divide the mixture evenly among the plates, drizzle each salad with 2 tablespoons of dressing, and enjoy!

PER SERVING

Calories: 485 | Calories From Fat: 279 | Total Fat: 31 g | Saturated Fat: 4.5 g | Cholesterol: 242 mg | Sodium: 636 mg | Carbs: 19.4 g | Dietary Fiber: 7.2 g | Net Carbs: 12.2 g | Sugars: 5.4 g | Protein: 32.2 g

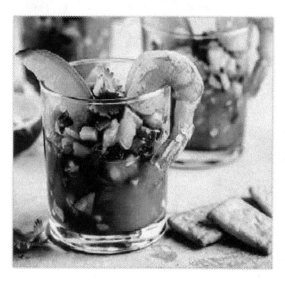

Sea Bass with Dijon Butter Sauce

Prep time: 5 minutes | Cook time: 20 minutes |Serves 3

- 2 tablespoons olive oil
- 2 sea bass fillets
- 1/4 teaspoon red pepper flakes, crushed
- Sea salt, to taste
- 1/3 teaspoon mixed peppercorns, crushed
- 3 tablespoons butter
- 1 tablespoon Dijon mustard
- 2 cloves garlic, minced
- 1 tablespoon fresh lime juice

1. Heat the olive oil in a skillet over medium-high heat.
2. Pat dry the sea bass fillets with paper towels. Now pan-fry the fish fillets for about 4 minutes on each side until flesh flakes easily and it is nearly opaque.
3. Season your fish with red pepper, salt, and mixed peppercorns.
4. To make the sauce, melt the 3 tablespoons of butter in a saucepan over low heat; stir in the Dijon mustard, garlic, and lime juice. Let it simmer for 2 minutes.
5. To serve, spoon the Dijon butter sauce over the fish fillets. Bon appétit!

PER SERVING

Calories: 314 | Fat: 23.2g | Carbs: 1.4g | Protein: 24.2g | Fiber: 0.3g

Creamed Monkfish Salad

Prep time: 5 minutes | Cook time: 20 minutes |Serves 5

- 2 pounds monkfish
- 1 bell pepper, sliced
- 1/2 cup radishes, sliced
- 1 red onion, chopped
- 1 garlic clove, minced
- 1 tablespoon balsamic vinegar
- 1/2 cup mayonnaise
- 1 teaspoon stone-ground mustard
- Flaky salt, to season

1. Pat the fish dry with paper towels and brush on both sides with nonstick cooking oil. Grill over medium-high heat, flipping halfway through for about 9 minutes or until opaque.
2. Flake the fish with a fork and toss with the remaining ingredients; gently toss to combine well.
3. Serve at room temperature or well-chilled. Bon appétit!

PER SERVING

Calories: 306 | Fat: 19.4g | Carbs: 3.8g | Protein: 27g | Fiber: 0.6g

Creole Fish Stew with Turkey Smoked Sausage
Prep time: 10 minutes | Cook time: 20 minutes |Serves 4

- 2 tablespoons butter, at room temperature
- 1 onion, chopped
- 2 cloves garlic, sliced
- 1 bell pepper, sliced
- 1 celery stalk, chopped
- 1 cup broccoli florets
- 4 ounces turkey smoked sausage, sliced
- Sea salt and ground black pepper, to taste
- 2 tomatoes, pureed
- 2 cups fish broth
- 1 teaspoon chili powder
- 1/4 teaspoon ground allspice
- 16 ounces haddock steak, cut into bite-sized chunks
- 2 tablespoons fresh coriander, minced
- 1 teaspoon Creole seasoning blend

1. Melt the butter in a heavy-bottomed pot over moderate heat. Now, sauté the onion, garlic, and pepper, for 2 minutes until just tender and aromatic.
2. Add in the celery, broccoli, turkey smoked sausage, salt, black pepper, pureed tomatoes, and broth. Bring to a rolling boil and immediately reduce the heat to simmer.
3. Add in the remaining ingredients, partially cover, and continue simmering for 15 minutes.
4. Ladle into soup bowls and serve immediately.

PER SERVING

Calories: 236 | Fat: 9.4g | Carbs: 6.1g | Protein: 27g | Fiber: 2.1g

Salmon Salad Cups
Prep time: 10 minutes | Cook time:5 minutes |Serves 4

- 12 ounces (340 g) canned salmon (no salt added)
- 3 tablespoons prepared horseradish
- 1 tablespoon chopped fresh dill
- 2 teaspoons lemon juice
- ½ teaspoon finely ground sea salt
- ½ teaspoon ground black pepper
- 12 butter lettuce leaves (from 1 head)
- ½ cup (105 g) mayonnaise

1. Place the salmon, horseradish, dill, lemon juice, salt, and pepper in a medium-sized bowl. Stir until the ingredients are fully incorporated.
2. Set the lettuce leaves on a serving plate. Fill each leaf with 2 tablespoons of the salmon salad mixture and top with 2 teaspoons of mayonnaise.

PER SERVING

Calories: 314 | Total Fat: 26.5 g | Sodium: 526 mg | Carbs: 4.4 g | Dietary Fiber: 1.1 g | Net Carbs: 3.3 g | Sugars: 1.8 g | Protein: 14.6 g

Marinated and Grilled Salmon
Prep time: 5 minutes | Cook time: 1 hour |Serves 4

- 4 (5-ounce) salmon steaks
- 2 cloves garlic, pressed
- 4 tablespoons olive oil
- 1 tablespoon Taco seasoning mix
- 2 tablespoons fresh lemon juice

1. Place all of the above ingredients in a ceramic dish; cover and let it marinate for 40 minutes in your refrigerator.
2. Place the salmon steaks onto a lightly oiled grill pan; place under the grill for 6 minutes.
3. Turn them over and cook for a further 5 to 6 minutes, basting with the reserved marinade; remove from the grill.
4. Serve immediately and enjoy!

PER SERVING

Calories: 331 | Fat: 21.4g | Carbs: 2.2g | Protein: 30.4g | Fiber: 0.4g

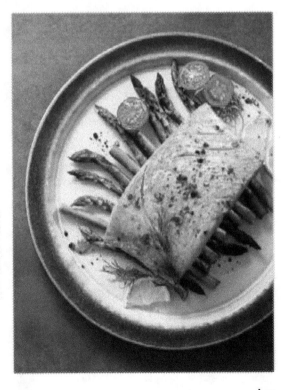

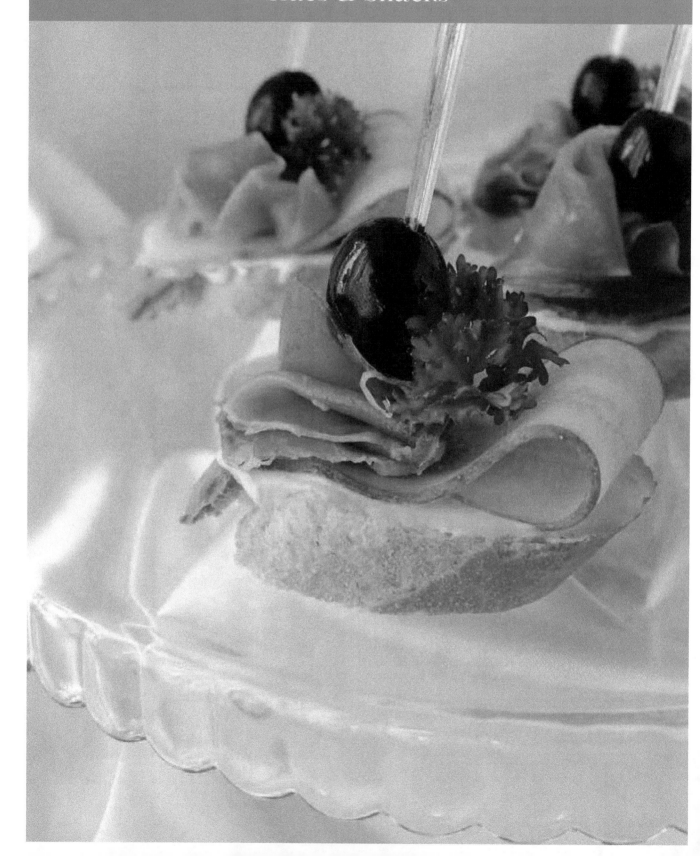

Chapter 8
Sides & Snacks

Sammies With Basil Mayo

Prep time: 10 minutes | Cook time:5 minutes |Serves 1

- Basil Mayo:
- ½ cup (105 g) mayonnaise
- 8 large fresh basil leaves, finely chopped
- 1 tablespoon lemon juice
- 1 clove garlic, minced
- ¼ teaspoon finely ground sea salt
- Pinch of ground black pepper
- Sammies:
- 1 small head iceberg lettuce
- 4 slices deli turkey
- 4 slices deli ham
- 1 medium Hass avocado, peeled, pitted, and sliced (about 4 oz/110 g of flesh)

1. Place the ingredients for the basil mayo in a small bowl and whisk to combine.
2. Cut the head of lettuce in half, then cut each half in half again so you have 4 wedges.
3. Set a lettuce wedge on its side on a plate and layer on 2 slices of turkey, 2 slices of ham, and half of the avocado slices. Top with half of the basil mayo, then set a second lettuce wedge on top, placing it so that the thick edge of the top wedge is aligned with the thin edge of the bottom wedge. (This will give your sandwich an even thickness, making it much easier to eat!)
4. Repeat with the remaining lettuce wedges, sandwich fixings, and basil mayo and enjoy.

PER SERVING

Calories: 653 | Calories From Fat: 514 | Total Fat: 57.1 g | Carbs: 16 g | Dietary Fiber: 6.4 g | Net Carbs: 9.6 g | Sugars: 5.4 g | Protein: 18.8 g

Keto Fat Bombs

Prep time: 5 minutes | Cook time: 1 hour | Serves 12

- 1 stick (½ cup) butter
- ½ cup crunchy almond butter
- 1 teaspoon vanilla extract
- ½ teaspoon cinnamon

1. Line a 12-cup muffin pan with paper liners.
2. In a small saucepan over medium-low heat, melt the butter and almond butter. Remove from the heat.
3. Add the vanilla and cinnamon, stirring until well combined.
4. Fill the muffin cups equally with the mixture.
5. Freeze for 30 minutes to 1 hour. Store in refrigerator.

PER SERVING

Calories: 199 | Fat: 19g | Saturated Fat: 5.5g | Protein: 5.4g | Carbohydrate: 4.1g | Fiber: 2.1g | Sodium: 54mg

Coconut Chocolate Bars

Prep time: 5 minutes | Cook time: 1 hour, 30 minutes | Serves 12

CRUST:

- 6 tablespoons cultured butter, melted (orghee)
- 2 cups almond flour
- 1½ tablespoons stevia (about 10 packets)
- Pinch of salt
- Coconut Layer:
- 2 cups unsweetened coconut flakes
- ⅔ cup full-fat coconut milk
- ¼ cup coconut oil, melted
- ¼ cup monk fruit syrup, maple flavored
- ¼ teaspoon almond extract
- Chocolate Layer:
- ½ cup coconut oil, melted
- ¼ cup plus 2 tablespoons monk fruit syrup, maple flavored
- ½ cup unsweetened cocoa powder

1. Preheat the oven to 350°F. Line an 8 x 8-inch baking pan with parchment paper.
2. Combine all the crust and press into the pan. Bake for 15 minutes. Remove from the oven and let cool.
3. To make the coconut layer, put all the in a food processor and pulse until fully combined. Pour on top of the crust layer and place in the refrigerator for 15 minutes.
4. To make the chocolate layer, warm the coconut oil and syrup in a small saucepan and stir well. Add the cocoa powder and stir until combined. Pour over the coconut layer and return the pan to the refrigerator for 30 minutes to 1 hour, or until set.
5. Cut and serve cold. Store in the refrigerator.

PER SERVING

Calories: 327 | Fat: 33.4g | Saturated Fat: 26.5g | Protein: 2.3g | Carbohydrate: 6.2g | Fiber: 3.9g | Sodium: 80mg

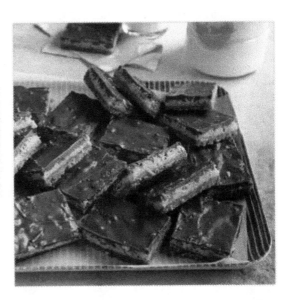

Keto Brownies

Prep time: 5 minutes | Cook time: 50 minutes | Serves 16

- ½ cup almond flour
- ¼ cup unsweetened cocoa powder
- ½ teaspoon sea salt
- ½ teaspoon baking powder
- 2 ounces unsweetened dark chocolate
- ½ cup coconut oil
- ½ cup monk fruit sweetener
- 3 large eggs, at room temperature
- ½ teaspoon vanilla extract

1. Preheat the oven to 350°F. Line an 8 x 8-inch baking pan with parchment paper.
2. In a medium bowl, mix together the flour, cocoa powder, salt, and baking powder.
3. In a double boiler or microwave, melt the dark chocolate and coconut oil together and stir until smooth. (If using the microwave, heat at 30-second intervals, stirring between intervals.)
4. In a large bowl, beat the sweetener, eggs, and vanilla together vigorously. Add the chocolate mixture and continue to mix.
5. Fold in the flour mixture and mix until the batter is smooth.
6. Pour the batter into the baking pan and bake for 20 minutes, or until a toothpick inserted into the center comes out clean. Cut into 16 brownies and serve. Store in the refrigerator.

PER SERVING

Calories: 139 | Fat: 13.1g | Saturated Fat: 9.3g | Protein: 3.2g | Carbohydrate: 10.9g | Fiber: 2.6g | Sodium: 73mg

Coffee Cake

Prep time: 5 minutes | Cook time: 55 minutes | Serves 9

CAKE:

- 2 tablespoons coconut oil, melted
- 1 large egg
- 1 teaspoon vanilla extract
- 1 teaspoon liquid stevia
- ½ cup coconut milk
- 1½ cups blanched almond flour
- 1 teaspoon cinnamon
- 2 teaspoons baking powder
- ½ teaspoon sea salt

TOPPING:

- ½ cup blanched almond flour
- 1½ tablespoons coconut oil, melted
- 5 drops liquid stevia
- 2 teaspoons cinnamon

1. Preheat the oven to 350°F. grease an 8 x 8-inch baking dish or loaf pan.
2. In a large bowl, combine the coconut oil, egg, vanilla extract, stevia, and coconut milk, and stir until well combined.

3. In a medium bowl, combine the almond flour, cinnamon, baking powder, and salt.
4. Add the dry to the wet and stir until smooth.
5. Pour the batter into the greased baking dish.
6. In a small bowl, mix the topping together and crumble over the cake.
7. Bake for 45 to 50 minutes. Remove from the oven, test doneness with a toothpick, let cool, and remove from the baking dish. Serve warm. Store in the refrigerator.

PER SERVING

Calories: 130 | Fat: 12.3g | Saturated Fat: 8.5g | Protein: 2.4g | Carbohydrate: 2.9g | Fiber: 1.4g | Sodium: 117mg

Keto Bread

Prep time: 5 minutes | Cook time: 40 minutes | Serves 10

- ¼ teaspoon cream of tartar
- 6 large egg whites
- 1½ cups almond flour
- 4 tablespoons butter, melted
- ¾ teaspoon baking soda
- 3 teaspoons apple cider vinegar
- 2 tablespoons coconut flour

1. Preheat the oven to 375°F. grease an 8 x 4-inch loaf pan.
2. In a medium bowl, combine the cream of tartar and the egg whites. Beat the egg whites with an electric mixer until they form soft peaks.
3. Put the almond flour, butter, baking soda, apple cider vinegar, and coconut flour in a food processor, and blend until well combined.
4. Remove the mixture to a large bowl and gently fold in the egg whites.
5. Pour the batter into the loaf pan and bake for 30 minutes.
6. Remove from the oven and let cool for 10 minutes. Store in the refrigerator.

PER SERVING

Calories: 44 | Fat: 3.5g | Saturated Fat: 1.6g | Protein: 1.8g | Carbohydrate: 1.6g | Fiber: 0.8g | Sodium: 73mg

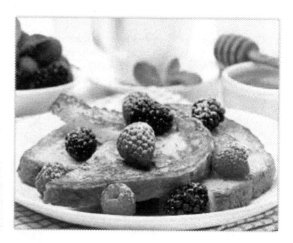

Keto Chocolate Chip Cookies

Prep time: 5 minutes | Cook time: 22 minutes | Serves 24

- 2 cups almond flour
- 1 scoop collagen protein
- ½ teaspoon baking powder
- ¼ teaspoon sea salt
- ½ cup coconut oil, melted
- ½ cup monk fruit sweetener
- 1 teaspoon pure vanilla extract
- 2 large eggs
- ½ cup unsweetened chocolate chips

1. Preheat the oven to 350°F. Line a baking sheet with parchment paper.
2. In a large bowl, mix together the almond flour, collagen | Protein: baking powder, and sea salt. Set aside.
3. In a small bowl, mix together the coconut oil, monk fruit sweetener, vanilla, and eggs.
4. Incorporate the coconut oil mixture into the flour mixture until a thick dough forms. Stir in the chocolate chips.
5. Scoop and roll the dough into 24 balls andgently flatten with the back of a spoon or your fingertips. Place them 2 inches apart on the prepared baking sheet.
6. Bake for 10 to 12 minutes. Remove from the sheet and allow to cool on a wire rack. Store in the refrigerator.

PER SERVING

Calories: 54 | Fat: 4.2g | Saturated Fat: 1.9g | Protein: 2.0g | Carbohydrate: 5.9g | Fiber: 0.9g | Sodium: 26mg

Keto Chocolate Frosty

Prep time: 5 minutes | Cook time: 35 minutes | Serves 1

- 1 cup full fat coconut milk
- 2 tablespoons cocoa powder
- 1 tablespoon almond butter
- 1 teaspoon vanilla extract
- 1 tablespoon stevia (about 5 packets)

1. In a medium bowl, whisk together all the with an electric hand mixer, stand mixer, or a hand-whisk for 30 seconds, or until the are fully incorporated, thick, and creamy.
2. Freeze for 30 minutes. Whisk again for smoothness and enjoy.

PER SERVING

Calories: 579 | Fat: 58.6g | Saturated Fat: 44.3g | Protein: 9.9g | Carbohydrate: 15.8g | Fiber: 4.8g | Sodium: 33mg

Vegan Keto Cheesecake

Prep time: 5 minutes | Cook time: 1 hour, 25 minutes | Serves 12

CRUST:

- 1½ cups almond flour
- 1 packet stevia
- 5 tablespoons coconut oil, melted
- 1 teaspoon pure vanilla extract

FILLING:

- 16 ounces cashew vegan cream cheese
- 1 cup unsweetened coconut yogurt
- 1 teaspoon lemon zest
- 1 teaspoon lemon juice
- 1 tablespoon stevia (about 5 packets)
- 2 tablespoons coconut oil, melted

1. Preheat the oven to 350°F.
2. In a small bowl, mix together the crust . Press into the bottom of a 9-inch springform pan and bake for 10 minutes. Remove and let cool.
3. In a medium bowl, whisk together all the filling until incorporated and creamy. Pour on top of the baked crust and freeze for about 1 hour. Once firm, it is ready to enjoy. Store in an airtight container in the refrigerator for up to 3 days.

PER SERVING

Calories: 328 | Fat: 29g | Saturated Fat: 20.2g | Protein: 8g | Carbohydrate: 11g | Fiber: 0.5g | Sodium: 166mg

Keto Deviled Eggs

Prep time: 5 minutes | Cook time: 18 minutes | Serves 6

- 12 large eggs
- ¼ cup avocado oil mayonnaise
- 1 tablespoon Dijon mustard
- 1 teaspoon apple cider vinegar
- 1 teaspoon dill pickle juice
- 1 teaspoon sea salt
- ½ teaspoon freshlyground black pepper
- Paprika, to taste

1. In a large pot, place the eggs in water to cover and bring to a boil over medium-high heat. Cover the pot and turn off the heat. Let the eggs sit for 8 minutes.
2. Remove the eggs with a slotted spoon and cool them in a large bowl of ice water.
3. When the eggs are cool, remove the shells and slice in half lengthwise. Carefully remove the yolks and put them in a medium mixing bowl.
4. Add the remaining , except the paprika, to the yolks and whisk together until blended.
5. Spoon or pipe the yolk mixture into each egg half.
6. Sprinkle with the paprika and enjoy. Store in the refrigerator.

PER SERVING

Calories: 98 | Fat: 8.1g | Saturated Fat: 1.9g | Protein: 5.6g | Carbohydrate: 0.5g | Fiber: 0.1g | Sodium: 270mg

Keto Fudge

Prep time: 5 minutes | Cook time: 3 hours | Serves 10

- 1 cup full-fat coconut cream
- ¼ cup powdered monk fruit sweetener
- 2 teaspoons vanilla extract
- 2 tablespoons butter, room temperature
- 1 cup stevia-sweetened dark chocolate chips

1. Line a loaf pan with parchment paper.
2. In a small saucepan over medium heat, bring the coconut cream, monk fruit sweetener, and vanilla to a simmer, stirring often. Simmer for 20 minutes, or until it has reduced by nearly half and has the consistency of condensed milk.
3. Reduce the heat to low and stir in the butter until it has melted.
4. Stir in the dark chocolate chips until they have melted.
5. Remove from the heat and pour into the prepared loaf pan. Place in the refrigerator for at least 2 hours, or until the fudge has set. Turn upside down on a wooden cutting board and pop out. Use a sharp, heavy knife to carefully cut 1-inch square pieces. Store in the refrigerator.

PER SERVING

Calories: 166 | Fat: 14.4g | Saturated Fat: 10.5g | Protein: 2.2g | Carbohydrate: 17.4g | Fiber: 3.7g | Sodium: 20mg

Lemon Coconut Cheesecake Fat Bombs

Prep time: 5 minutes | Cook time: 1 hour, 10 minutes | Serves 12

- 4 ounces full-fat cream cheese, softened
- ¼ cup coconut butter
- 3 tablespoons coconut flour
- 2 tablespoons monk fruit powdered sweetener
- Zest of 1 lemon
- Juice of ½ lemon
- ½ teaspoon vanilla extract

1. Line a baking sheet with parchment paper.
2. In a small bowl, beat the cream cheese and coconut butter together with a handheld or stand mixer.
3. Add the remaining and beat on medium speed until well combined.
4. Place the dough in the refrigerator to chill for 30 minutes.
5. Roll the dough into balls using 2 tablespoons of dough. Set the balls on the baking sheet. Repeat until all the dough is used.
6. Place the baking sheet in the freezer for 30 minutes, or until hard. Store in an airtight container in the freezer or in the refrigerator.

PER SERVING

Calories: 131 | Fat: 11.5g | Saturated Fat: 3.5g | Protein: 5.1g | Carbohydrate: 6.8g | Fiber: 1.5g | Sodium: 52mg

Low-Carb Burger

Prep time: 5 minutes | Cook time: 25 minutes | Serves 2

- 1 pound (450 grams) ground beef (preferably lean)
- 1/4 cup almond flour
- 1/4 cup grated Parmesan cheese
- 1 small onion, finely chopped
- 1 clove garlic, minced
- 1 tablespoon Worcestershire sauce
- Salt and pepper to taste
- Lettuce leaves
- Sliced tomatoes
- Sliced avocado
- Condiments of your choice (sugar-free ketchup, mustard, etc.)

1. Preheat your grill or stovetop pan over medium-high heat.
2. In a mixing bowl, combine the ground beef, almond flour, grated Parmesan cheese, chopped onion, minced garlic, Worcestershire sauce, salt, and pepper. Mix well until all ingredients are evenly incorporated.
3. Divide the mixture into equal portions and shape them into burger patties. Make sure the patties are slightly larger than the size of your burger buns, as they will shrink during cooking.
4. Place the burger patties on the grill or stovetop pan and cook for about 4-5 minutes per side, or until they reach your desired level of doneness.
5. Once the burgers are cooked, remove them from the heat and let them rest for a few minutes.
6. Assemble your low-carb burger by placing a burger patty on a lettuce leaf. Top it with sliced tomatoes, avocado, and any other desired toppings. Add condiments such as sugar-free ketchup or mustard if desired.
7. Serve your delicious low-carb burger with a side of salad or steamed vegetables.

PER SERVING

Calories: 400-450|Protein: 25-30 grams|Fat: 25-30 grams|Carbohydrates: 5-7 grams|Fiber: 2-3 grams

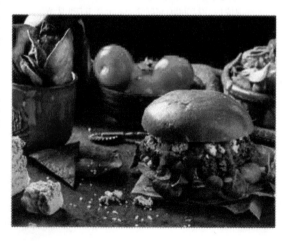

Roasted Mixed Nuts

Prep time: 5 minutes | Cook time: 20 minutes | Serves 4

- 1 cup raw pecans
- 1 cup raw cashews
- 1 cup raw almonds
- 1 cup raw walnuts
- 3 tablespoons coconut oil, melted
- 1 tablespoon sea salt
- 1 teaspoon cayenne pepper (optional)

1. Preheat the oven to 350°F. Line a baking sheet with parchment paper.
2. Toss all the together in a mixing bowl until the nuts are evenly coated with oil.
3. Spread the nuts out on the baking sheet and bake for 14 to 16 minutes, until lightly browned and fragrant. Remove and let cool. Store in aglass container at room temperature.

PER SERVING

Calories: 674 | Fat: 62.2g | Saturated Fat: 15.7g | Protein: 18.6g | Carbohydrate: 20.6g | Fiber: 7g | Sodium: 1,411mg

Spicy Roasted Pumpkin Seeds

Prep time: 5 minutes | Cook time: 10 minutes | Serves 8

- 4 tablespoons coconut oil
- 2 cups raw pumpkin seeds
- 4 teaspoons Tabasco sauce
- ½ teaspoon cayenne pepper

1. Line a baking sheet with parchment paper.
2. Heat the oil in a large pan over medium heat.
3. Add the pumpkin seeds and sauté for 2 to 3 minutes, or until they start to pop and turngolden brown.
4. Add the Tabasco and cayenne, toss, and continue to cook for 1 minute.
5. Transfer to the baking sheet, carefully spread the seeds out in a single layer, and let cool before serving. Store in aglass container at room temperature.

PER SERVING

Calories: 246 | Fat: 22.7g | Saturated Fat: 8.9g | Protein: 8.5g | Carbohydrate: 6.2g | Fiber: 1.4g | Sodium: 21mg

Broccoli Tabbouleh With Greek Chicken Thighs

Prep time: 15 minutes | Cook time:30 minutes |Serves 6

GREEK CHICKEN THIGHS:

- 6 bone-in, skin-on chicken thighs (about 2½ lbs/1.2 kg)
- ¼ cup (60 ml) avocado oil
- 2 tablespoons lemon juice
- 2 cloves garlic, minced
- 2 teaspoons chopped fresh rosemary
- 2 teaspoons dried thyme leaves
- 1 teaspoon dried oregano leaves
- Tabbouleh:
- ½ cup (120 ml) avocado oil
- ¼ cup (60 ml) lemon juice
- 4 cloves garlic, minced
- 4 green onions, finely chopped
- 3 tablespoons finely chopped fresh mint leaves
- ½ teaspoon finely ground sea salt
- 6 cups (425 g) broccoli florets
- 3 medium tomatoes, diced
- 1 cucumber, seeded and diced
- 1 bunch fresh parsley, finely chopped

1. Place the chicken thighs, oil, lemon juice, garlic, rosemary, thyme, and oregano in a dish. Turn the thighs in the mixture to coat, then cover and place in the refrigerator to marinate for 4 hours or overnight.
2. When ready to cook the chicken, preheat the oven to 350°F (177°C). Line a rimmed baking sheet with parchment paper.
3. Place the chicken on the lined baking sheet and bake for 25 to 30 minutes, until the internal temperature reaches 165°F (74°C) and the juices run clear.
4. Meanwhile, make the tabbouleh: Place the oil, lemon juice, garlic, green onions, mint, and salt in a large mixing bowl. Mix until incorporated.
5. Place half of the broccoli florets in a blender or food processor. Pulse until the pieces are ⅛ inch (3 mm) in size. Transfer the pieces to the large mixing bowl and repeat with the remaining broccoli florets.
6. Add the tomatoes, cucumber, and parsley to the bowl with the other tabbouleh ingredients and toss until fully incorporated.
7. Serve the tabbouleh with the chicken thighs.

PER SERVING

Calories: 779 | Calories From Fat: 592 | Total Fat: 65.8 g | Saturated Fat: 14.3 g | Cholesterol: 196 mg | Sodium: 300 mg | Carbs: 11.2 g | Dietary Fiber: 4.1 g | Net Carbs: 7.1 g | Sugars: 4.1 g | Protein: 35.5 g

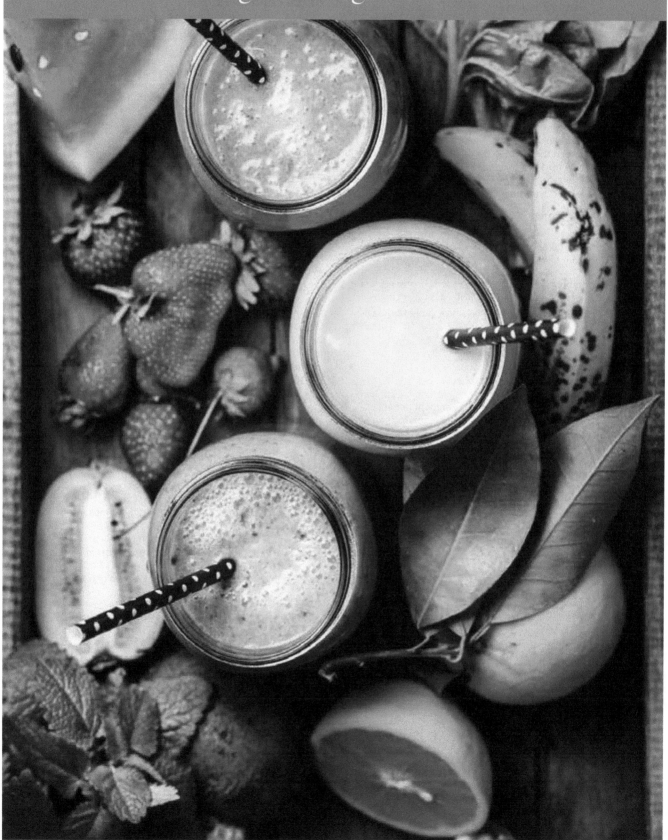

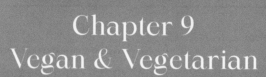
Chapter 9
Vegan & Vegetarian

Cauliflower, Cheese & Collard Greens Waffles

Prep time: 45 minutes | Cook time: 5 minutes | Serves 4

- 2 green onions
- 1 tbsp olive oil
- 2 eggs
- 1/3 cup Parmesan cheese
- 1 cup collard greens
- 1 cup mozzarella cheese
- ½ cauliflower head
- 1 tsp garlic powder
- 1 tbsp sesame seeds
- 2 tsp thyme, chopped

1. Place the chopped cauliflower in the food processor and process until rice is formed. Add collard greens, spring onions, and thyme to the food processor. Pulse until smooth. Transfer to a bowl.
2. Stir in the rest of the ingredients and mix to combine.
3. Heat waffle iron and spread the mixture onto the iron. Cook following the manufacturer's instructions.

PER SERVING

Cal: 283 | Net Carbs: 3.5g | Fat: 20.3g | Protein 16g

Easy Chopped Salad

Prep time: 10 minutes | Cook time: 5 minutes | Serves 1

- 1 small head romaine lettuce, chopped
- 8 cherry or grape tomatoes, halved
- ½ cucumber, seeded and chopped
- 1 celery stick, chopped
- ¼ cup (45 g) pitted black olives, chopped
- 2 tablespoons diced red onions
- 2 tablespoons chopped fresh mint
- ¼ cup (60 ml) vinaigrette of choice

1. Place the lettuce in a large serving bowl.
2. Top with the remaining salad ingredients, then drizzle with the vinaigrette and enjoy.

PER SERVING

Calories: 476 | Calories From Fat: 378 | Total Fat: 42 g | Saturated Fat: 5.1 g | Cholesterol: 0 mg | Sodium: 608 mg | Carbs: 18 g | Dietary Fiber: 6.5 g | Net Carbs: 11.5 g | Sugars: 7.1 g | Protein: 6.5 g

German No-Tato Salad

Prep time: 10 minutes | Cook time: 10 minutes | Serves 5

- 2 medium rutabaga (2 lbs/910 g), peeled
- 1 teaspoon finely ground sea salt
- 1 small red onion, finely diced
- 4 green onions, sliced
- 1 tablespoon Dijon mustard
- 1 teaspoon erythritol
- ¾ teaspoon ground black pepper
- For Serving:
- 1 tablespoon plus 2 teaspoons Dijon mustard
- 1 tablespoon plus 2 teaspoons mayonnaise
- 10 ounces (285 g) thinly sliced deli ham or other meat of choice

1. Cut the rutabaga into ½-inch (1.25-cm) cubes, place in a large saucepan, cover completely with water, and add the salt. Cover with the lid, bring to a boil over high heat, then reduce the heat to a simmer and cook for 10 minutes, or until fork-tender.
2. Meanwhile, place the remaining ingredients in a large salad bowl. Once the rutabaga is cooked, drain completely and transfer to the salad bowl. Toss to combine, then divide among 5 plates.
3. Serve the ham slices alongside the salad with 2 teaspoons of the mustard sauce.

PER SERVING

Calories: 296 | Calories From Fat: 167 | Total Fat: 18.8 g | Saturated Fat: 3.2 g | Cholesterol: 33 mg | Sodium: 1377 mg | Carbs: 19 g | Dietary Fiber: 5 g | Net Carbs: 14 g | Sugars: 10 g | Protein: 14 g

Stuffed Mushrooms

Prep time: 30 minutes | Cook time: 35 minutes | Serves 4

- 2 tbsp olive oil
- ¼ tsp chili flakes
- 1 cup gorgonzola, crumbled
- 1 garlic clove, minced
- 1 lb mushrooms, stems removed
- Salt and black pepper, to taste
- ¼ cup walnuts, toasted, chopped
- 2 tbsp parsley, chopped

1. Put to a pan over medium heat and warm the olive oil. Sauté garlic and onion, until soft, for about 5 minutes. Sprinkle with black pepper and salt, and remove to a bowl.
2. Add in walnuts and gorgonzola cheese and stir until heated through. Divide the filling among the mushroom caps and set on a greased baking sheet. Bake for 30 minutes at 360F and remove to a wire rack to cool slightly. Add fresh parsley and serve.

PER SERVING

Cal: 139 | Fat 11.2g | Net Carbs: 7.4g | Protein 4.8g

Speckled Salad

Prep time: 10 minutes | Cook time:5 minutes |Serves 1

DRESSING:

- ¼ cup (60 ml) lemon juice
- 2 tablespoons plus 2 teaspoons olive oil
- 1 teaspoon peeled and minced fresh ginger root
- 2 cloves garlic, minced
- Pinch of finely ground sea salt
- Pinch of ground black pepper

SALAD:

- 1 cup (60 g) destemmed kale leaves, roughly chopped
- 3 cups (85 g) mixed salad greens
- ¼ cup (38 g) hulled hemp seeds
- Handful of fresh cilantro leaves, chopped
- Handful of fresh flat-leaf parsley leaves, chopped
- Handful of fresh mint leaves, chopped

1. Place the dressing ingredients in a large salad bowl and stir until blended.
2. For the salad, rinse the chopped kale under hot water for 30 seconds or so to soften it up and make it easier to digest, then dry well. Add the dried kale leaves along with the rest of the salad ingredients to the bowl with the dressing. Toss to coat, then serve.

PER SERVING

Calories: 496 | Calories From Fat: 367 | Total Fat: 40.8 g | Saturated Fat: 6 g | Cholesterol: 0 mg | Sodium: 187 mg | Carbs: 23 g | Dietary Fiber: 5.6 g | Net Carbs: 17.4 g | Sugars: 4.4 g | Protein: 9.3 g

Kale Salad With Spicy Lime-Tahini Dressing

Prep time: 15 minutes | Cook time:5 minutes |Serves 4

DRESSING:

- ½ cup (120 ml) avocado oil
- ¼ cup (60 ml) lime juice
- ¼ cup (60 ml) tahini
- 2 cloves garlic, minced
- 1 jalapeño pepper, seeded and finely diced
- Handful of fresh cilantro leaves, chopped
- ½ teaspoon ground cumin
- ½ teaspoon finely ground sea salt
- ¼ teaspoon red pepper flakes

SALAD:

- 6 cups (360 g) destemmed kale leaves, roughly chopped
- 12 radishes, thinly sliced
- 1 green bell pepper, sliced
- 1 medium Hass avocado, peeled, pitted, and cubed (about 4 oz/110 g of flesh)
- ¼ cup (30 g) hulled pumpkin seeds

1. Make the dressing: Place the dressing ingredients in a medium-sized bowl and whisk to combine.

Set aside.

2. Make the salad: Rinse the kale under hot water for about 30 seconds to soften it and make it easier to digest. Dry the kale well, then place it in a large salad bowl. Add the remaining salad ingredients and toss to combine.
3. Divide the salad evenly among 4 bowls. Drizzle each bowl with ¼ cup (60 ml) of the dressing and serve.

PER SERVING

Calories: 517 | Calories From Fat: 423 | Total Fat: 47 g | Saturated Fat: 6 g | Cholesterol: 0 mg | Sodium: 373 mg | Carbs: 20.9 g | Dietary Fiber: 9.4 g | Net Carbs: 11.5 g | Sugars: 3.9 g | Protein: 10.7 g

Oven-Roasted Asparagus with Romesco Sauce

Prep time: 15 minutes | Cook time: 9 minutes |Serves 4

- 1 pound asparagus spears, trimmed
- 2 tbsp olive oil
- Salt and black pepper, to taste
- ½ tsp paprika
- Romesco sauce
- 2 red bell peppers, roasted
- 2 tsp olive oil
- 2 tbsp almond flour
- ½ cup scallions, chopped
- 1 garlic clove, minced
- 1 tbsp lemon juice
- ½ tsp chili pepper
- Salt and black pepper, to taste
- 2 tbsp rosemary, chopped

1. In a food processor, pulse together the bell peppers, salt, black pepper, garlic, lemon juice, scallions, almond flour, 2 tsp of olive oil and chili pepper. Mix evenly and set aside.
2. Preheat oven to 390 F and line a baking sheet with parchment paper. Add asparagus spears to the baking sheet. Toss with 2 tbsp of olive oil, paprika, black pepper, and salt. Bake until cooked through for 9 minutes. Transfer to a serving plate, pour the sauce over and garnish with rosemary to serve.

PER SERVING

Cal: 145 | Fat 11g | Net Carbs: 5.9g | Protein 4.1g

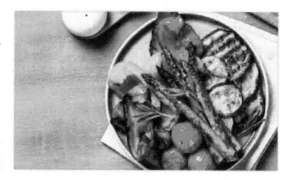

Antipasto Salad

Prep time: 10 minutes | Cook time:5 minutes |Serves 4

- 1 (12-oz/340-g) jar roasted red peppers, drained and roughly chopped
- 1 (6½-oz/185-g) jar marinated artichoke quarters, drained and roughly chopped
- 1 (4-oz/113-g) can sliced cremini mushrooms, drained
- 4 ounces (115 g) salami, sliced
- 3 tablespoons capers, drained
- ¾ cup (210 ml) vinaigrette of choice

1. Place all the ingredients in a large mixing bowl.
2. Toss to coat, then serve.

PER SERVING

Calories: 433 | Total Fat: 38.9 g | Carbs: 13.5 g | Fiber: 4.4 g | Net Carbs: 9.1 g | Sugars: 5 g | Protein: 7.3 g

Spinach & Feta Frittata

Prep time: 35 minutes | Cook time: 25 minutes | Serves 4

- 5 ounces spinach
- 8 ounces feta cheese, crumbled
- 1 pint cherry tomatoes, halved
- 10 eggs
- 3 tbsp olive oil
- 4 scallions, diced
- Salt and black pepper to taste

1. Preheat your oven to 350 F. Drizzle the oil in a 2-quart casserole and place in the oven until heated.
2. In a bowl, whisk the eggs along with the pepper and salt until thoroughly combined. Stir in the spinach, feta cheese, and scallions. Pour the mixture into the casserole, top with the cherry tomatoes, and place back in the oven. Bake for 25 minutes until your frittata is set in the middle.
3. When done, remove the casserole from the oven, and run a spatula around the edges of the frittata, slide it onto a warm platter. Cut the frittata into wedges, and serve with salad.

PER SERVING

Cal: 461 | Net Carbs: 6g | Fat: 35g | Protein 26g

Stuffed Mushrooms

Prep time: 30 minutes | Cook time: 35 minutes |Serves 4

- 2 tbsp olive oil
- ¼ tsp chili flakes
- 1 cup gorgonzola, crumbled
- 1 onion, chopped
- 1 garlic clove, minced
- 1 lb mushrooms, stems removed
- Salt and black pepper, to taste
- ¼ cup walnuts, toasted, chopped
- 2 tbsp parsley, chopped

1. Put to a pan over medium heat and warm the olive oil. Sauté garlic and onion, until soft, for about 5 minutes. Sprinkle with black pepper and salt, and remove to a bowl.
2. Add in walnuts and gorgonzola cheese and stir until heated through. Divide the filling among the mushroom caps and set on a greased baking sheet. Bake for 30 minutes at 360F and remove to a wire rack to cool slightly. Add fresh parsley and serve.

PER SERVING

Cal: 139 | Fat 11.2g | Net Carbs: 7.4g | Protein 4.8g

Zucchini Pasta Salad

Prep time: 5 minutes | Cook time:5 minutes |Serves 4

- 4 medium zucchinis, spiral sliced
- 12 ounces (340 g) pitted black olives, cut in half lengthwise
- 1 pint (290 g) cherry tomatoes, cut in half lengthwise
- ½ cup (75 g) pine nuts
- ¼ cup plus 2 tablespoons (55 g) sesame seeds
- ⅔ cup (160 ml) creamy Italian dressing or other creamy salad dressing of choice

1. Place all the ingredients in a large mixing bowl.
2. Toss to coat, then divide evenly between 4 serving plates or bowls.

PER SERVING

Calories: 562 | Calories From Fat: 471 | Total Fat: 53 g | Carbs: 22 g | Dietary Fiber: 8.5 g | Net Carbs: 13.5 g | Sugars: 6.7 g | Protein: 8.9 g

Tofu & Vegetable Stir-Fry

Prep time: 10 minutes| Cook time: 8 minutes | Serves 4

- 2 tbsp olive oil
- 1 ½ cups extra firm tofu, cubed
- 1 ½ tbsp flax seed meal
- Salt and black pepper, to taste
- 1 garlic clove, minced
- 1 tbsp soy sauce, sugar-free
- ½ head broccoli, break into florets
- 1 tsp onion powder
- 1 cup mushrooms, sliced
- 1 tbsp sesame seeds

1. In a bowl, add onion powder, tofu, salt, soy sauce, black pepper, flaxseed, and garlic. Toss the mixture to coat and allow to marinate for 20-30 minutes.
2. In a pan, warm oil over medium heat, add in broccoli, mushrooms and tofu mixture and stir-fry for 6-8 minutes. Serve sprinkled with sesame seeds.

PER SERVING

Cal: 423 | Fat 31g | Net Carbs: 7.3g | Protein 25g

Roasted Cauliflower Gratin

Prep time: 21 minutes | Cook time: 18 minutes |Serves 4

- 1/3 cup butter
- 2 tbsp melted butter
- 1 onion, chopped
- 2 heads cauliflower, cut into florets
- Salt and black pepper to taste
- ¼ cup almond milk
- ½ cup almond flour
- 1½ cups cheddar cheese, grated
- 1 tbsp ground almonds
- 1 tbsp parsley, chopped

1. Steam the cauliflower in salted water for 4-5 minutes. Drain and set aside.
2. Melt the 1/3 cup of butter in a saucepan over medium heat and sauté the onion for 3
3. minutes. Add the cauliflower, season with salt and black pepper and mix in almond milk.
4. Simmer for 3 minutes.
5. Mix the remaining melted butter with the almond flour. Stir into the cauliflower as well as half of the cheese. Sprinkle the top with the remaining cheese and ground almonds, and bake for 10 minutes until golden brown on the top. Serve sprinkled with parsley.

PER SERVING

Cal: 455 | Fat: 38.3g | Net Carbs: 6.5g | Protein 16.3g

Basil Spinach & Zucchini Lasagna

Prep time: 40 minutes | Cook time: 35 minutes |Serves 4

- 2 zucchinis, sliced
- Salt and black pepper to taste
- 2 cups feta cheese
- 2 cups mozzarella cheese, shredded
- 3 cups tomato sauce
- 1 cup spinach
- tbsp basil, chopped

1. Mix the feta, mozzarella cheese, salt, and black pepper to evenly combine and spread ¼ cup of the mixture at the bottom of a greased baking dish. Layer 1/3 of the zucchini slices on top, spread 1 cup of tomato sauce over and scatter a 1/3 cup of spinach on top.
2. Repeat the layering process two more times to exhaust the ingredients while making sure to layer with the last ¼ cup of cheese mixture finally. Bake for 35 minutes until the cheese has a nice golden brown color. Remove the dish, sit for 5 minutes and serve sprinkled with basil.

PER SERVING

Cal: 411 | Fat: 41.3g | Net Carbs: 3.2g | Protein 6.5g

Keto Tortilla Wraps with Vegetables

Prep time: 10 minutes | Cook time: 9 minutes |Serves 2

- 2 tsp olive oil
- 2 low carb tortillas
- 1 green onion, sliced
- 1 bell pepper, sliced
- ¼ tsp hot chili powder
- 1 large avocado, sliced
- 1 cup cauli rice
- Salt and black pepper to taste
- ¼ cup sour cream
- 1 tbsp Mexican salsa
- 1 tbsp cilantro, chopped

1. Warm the olive oil in a skillet and sauté the green onion and bell pepper until they start to brown on the edges, for about 4 minutes; remove to a bowl. To the same pan, add in the cauli rice and stir-fry for 4-5 minutes. Combine with the onion and bell pepper mixture, season with salt, black pepper, and chili powder. Let cool for a few minutes.
2. Add in avocado, sour cream, and Mexican salsa and stir. Top with cilantro. Fold in the sides of each tortilla, and roll them in and over the filling to be enclosed. Wrap with foil, cut in halves, and serve.

PER SERVING

Cal: 373 | Fat: 31.2g | Net Carbs: 8.6g | Protein 7.6g

Steamed Bok Choy with Thyme & Garlic

Prep time: 25 minutes | Cook time: 8 minutes |Serves 4

- 2 pounds Bok choy, sliced
- 2 tbsp coconut oil
- 2 tbsp soy sauce, sugar-free
- 1 tsp garlic, minced
- ½ tsp thyme, chopped
- ½ tsp red pepper flakes, crushed
- Salt and black pepper, to the taste

1. In a pot, steam bok choy in salted water over medium heat, for 6 minutes; drain and set aside. Place a pan over medium heat and warm the coconut oil. Add in garlic and cook until soft.
2. Stir in the bok choy, red pepper, soy sauce, black pepper, salt, and thyme and cook until everything is heated through, for about 1-2 minutes.

PER SERVING

Cal: 132 | Fat 9.5g | Net Carbs: 3.5g | Protein 4.9g

Broccoli Ginger Soup

Prep time: 5 minutes | Cook time:25 minutes |Serves 4

- 3 tablespoons coconut oil or avocado oil
- 1 small white onion, sliced
- 2 cloves garlic, minced
- 5 cups (420 g) broccoli florets
- 1 (13½-oz/400-ml) can full-fat coconut milk
- 1½ cups (355 ml) chicken bone broth
- 1 (2-in/5-cm) piece fresh ginger root, peeled and minced
- 1½ teaspoons turmeric powder
- ¾ teaspoon finely ground sea salt
- ⅓ cup (55 g) collagen peptides (optional)
- ¼ cup (40 g) sesame seeds

1. Melt the oil in a large frying pan over medium heat. Add the onion and garlic and cook until translucent, about 10 minutes.
2. Add the broccoli, coconut milk, broth, ginger, turmeric, and salt. Cover and cook for 15 minutes, or until the broccoli is tender.
3. Transfer the broccoli mixture to a blender or food processor. Add the collagen, if using, and blend until smooth.
4. Divide among 4 bowls, top each bowl with 1 tablespoon of sesame seeds, and enjoy!

PER SERVING

Calories: 344 | Calories From Fat: 241 | Total Fat: 26.8 g | Carbs: 12.4 g | Dietary Fiber: 4.5 g | Net Carbs: 7.9 g | Sugars: 2.9 g | Protein: 13.3 g

Spicy Cauliflower Falafel

Prep time: 15 minutes | Cook time: 5 minutes |Serves 4

- 4 tbsp olive oil
- 1 head cauliflower, cut into florets
- 1/3 cup silvered ground almonds
- ½ tsp ground cumin
- 1 tsp parsley, chopped
- Salt to taste
- 1 tsp chili pepper
- 3 tbsp coconut flour
- 4 eggs

1. Blitz the cauliflower in a food processor until a grain meal consistency is formed. Transfer to a bowl, add in the ground almonds, ground cumin, parsley, salt, chili pepper, and coconut flour, and mix until evenly combined.
2. Beat the eggs in a bowl and mix with the cauli mixture. Shape ¼ cup each into patties and set aside.
3. Warm olive oil in a frying pan over medium heat and fry the patties for 5 minutes on each side to be firm and browned. Remove onto a wire rack to cool, share into serving plates, and serve.

PER SERVING

Cal: 343 | Fat: 31.2g | Net Carbs: 3.7g | Protein 8.5g

Roasted Tomatoes with Vegan Cheese Crust

Prep time: 15 minutes | Cook time: 10 minutes |Serves 4

- 3 tomatoes, sliced
- 2 tbsp olive oil
- ½ cup pepitas seeds
- 1 tbsp nutritional yeast
- Salt and black pepper, to taste
- 1 tsp garlic puree
- 2 tbsp parsley. chopped

1. Preheat oven to 380 F and grease a baking pan with olive oil. Drizzle olive oil over the tomatoes.
2. In a food processor, add pepitas seeds, nutritional yeast, garlic puree, salt and pepper, and pulse until the desired consistency is attained. Press the mixture firmly onto each slice of tomato. Set the tomato slices on the prepared baking pan and bake for 10 minutes. Serve sprinkled with parsley.

PER SERVING

Cal: 165 | Fat 14.7g | Net Carbs: 3.2g | Protein 6.2g

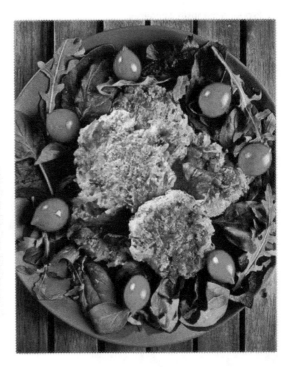

Tofu & Hazelnut Loaded Zucchini

Prep time: 50 minutes | Cook time: 42 minutes |Serves 4

- 2 tbsp olive oil
- 12 ounces firm tofu, crumbled
- 2 garlic cloves, pressed
- ½ cup onions, chopped
- 2 cups crushed tomatoes
- ¼ tsp dried oregano
- Salt and black pepper to taste
- ¼ tsp chili pepper
- 2 zucchinis, cut into halves, scoop out the insides ¼ cup hazelnuts, chopped
- 2 tbsp cilantro, chopped

1. Sauté onion, garlic, and tofu in olive oil for 5 minutes until softened. Place in scooped zucchini flesh, 1 cup of tomatoes, oregano, and chili pepper. Season with salt, and pepper and cook for 6 minutes.
2. Preheat oven to 390 F. Pour the remaining tomatoes in a baking dish. Spoon the tofu mixture into the zucchini shells. Arrange the zucchini boats in the baking dish. Bake for about 30 minutes. Sprinkle with hazelnuts and continue baking for 5 to 6 more minutes.
3. Scatter with cilantro to serve.

PER SERVING

Cal: 234 | Fat 18.3g | Net Carbs: 5.9g | Protein 12.5g

Veggie Noodles with Avocado Sauce

Prep time: 15 minutes | Cook time: 8 minutes |Serves 4

- ½ pound pumpkin, spiralized
- ½ pound bell peppers, spiralized
- 2 tbsp olive oil
- 2 avocados, chopped
- 1 lemon, juiced and zested
- 2 tbsp sesame oil
- 2 tbsp cilantro, chopped
- 1 onion, chopped
- 1 jalapeño pepper, deveined and minced
- Salt and black pepper, to taste
- 2 tbsp pumpkin seeds

1. Toast pumpkin seeds in a dry skillet, stirring frequently for a minute; set aside. Add in oil and sauté bell peppers and pumpkin for 8 minutes. Remove to a serving platter.
2. Combine avocados, sesame oil, onion, jalapeño pepper, lemon juice, and lemon zest in a food processor and pulse to obtain a creamy mixture. Adjust the seasoning and pour over the vegetable noodles, top with the pumpkin seeds and serve.

PER SERVING

Cal: 673 | Fat 59g | Net Carbs: 9.8g | Protein 22.9g

Fresh Coconut Milk Shake with Blackberries

Prep time: 5 minutes | Cook time: 5 minutes |Serves 2

- ½ cup water
- 1 ½ cups coconut milk
- 2 cups fresh blackberries
- ¼ tsp vanilla extract
- 1 tbsp vegan protein powder

1. In a blender, combine all the ingredients and blend well until you attain a uniform and creamy consistency. Divide in glasses and serve!

PER SERVING

Cal: 253 | Fat 22g | Net Carbs: 5.6g | Protein 3.3g

Strawberry & Spinach Salad with Goat Cheese

Prep time: 25 minutes | Cook time: 25 minutes | Serves 2

- 4 cups spinach
- 4 strawberries, sliced
- ½ cup almonds, flaked
- 1 ½ cups hard goat cheese, grated
- 4 tbsp raspberry vinaigrette
- Salt and black pepper to taste

1. Preheat your oven to 400 F. Arrange the grated goat cheese in two circles on two pieces of parchment paper. Place in the oven, and bake for 10 minutes.
2. Find two same bowls, place them upside down, and carefully put the parchment paper on top of them, to give the cheese a bowl-like shape. Let cool that way for 15 minutes. Divide the spinach between the bowls. Drizzle the vinaigrette over. Top with almonds and strawberries.

PER SERVING

Cal: 645 | Net Carbs: 5.8g | Fat: 54g | Protein 33g

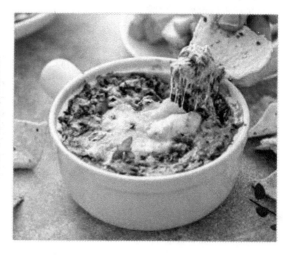

Balsamic Vegetables with Feta & Almonds

Prep time: 45 minutes | Cook time: 40 minutes |Serves 4

- 4 tbsp olive oil
- 1 red bell pepper, sliced
- 1 green bell pepper, sliced
- 1 orange bell pepper, sliced
- ½ head broccoli, cut into florets
- 2 zucchinis, sliced
- 8 white pearl onions, peeled
- 2 garlic cloves, halved
- 2 thyme sprigs, chopped
- 1 tsp dried sage, crushed
- 2 tbsp balsamic vinegar
- Sea salt and cayenne pepper, to taste
- 1 cup feta cheese, crumbled
- ½ cup almonds, toasted and chopped

1. Preheat oven to 375 F. Mix all vegetables with olive oil, seasonings, and balsamic vinegar; shake well. Spread the vegetables out in a baking dish and roast in the oven for 40 minutes or until tender, flipping once halfway through.
2. Remove from the oven to a serving plate. Scatter the feta cheese and almonds all over and serve.

PER SERVING

Cal: 276 | Fat 23.3g | Net Carbs: 7.9g | Protein 8.1g

Tasty Tofu & Swiss Chard Dip

Prep time: 10 minutes | Cook time: 6 minutes |Serves 4

- 2 tbsp mayonnaise
- 2 cups Swiss chard
- ½ cup tofu, pressed, crumbled
- ¼ cup almond milk
- 1 tsp nutritional yeast
- 1 garlic clove, minced
- 2 tbsp olive oil
- Salt and pepper to taste
- ½ tsp paprika
- ½ tsp mint leaves, chopped

1. Fill a pot with salted water and boil Swiss chard over medium heat for 5-6 minutes, until wilted. Puree the remaining ingredients, except for the mayonnaise, in a food processor.
2. Season with salt and black pepper. Stir in the Swiss chard and mayonnaise to get a homogeneous mixture.

PER SERVING

Cal: 136 | Fat: 11g | Net Carbs: 6.3g | Protein: 3.1g

Cauliflower-Based Waffles with Zucchini & Cheese

Prep time: 45 minutes | Cook time: 15 minutes |Serves 3

- 2 green onions
- 1 tbsp olive oil
- 2 eggs
- 1/3 cup Parmesan cheese
- 1 cup zucchini, shredded
- 1 cup mozzarella cheese, grated
- ½ head cauliflower
- 1 tsp garlic powder
- 1 tbsp sesame seeds
- 2 tsp thyme, chopped

1. Chop the cauliflower into florets, toss the pieces a the food processor and pulse until rice is formed. Remove to a clean kitchen towel and press to eliminate excess moisture. Return to the food processor and add zucchini, spring onions, and thyme; pulse until smooth and transfer to a bowl.
2. Stir in the rest of the ingredients and mix to combine. Leave to rest for 10 minutes. Heat waffle iron and spread in the mixture, evenly. Cook until golden brown, for about 5 minutes.

PER SERVING

Cal: 336 | Fat: 21g | Net Carbs: 7.2g | Protein 32.6g

Tofu & Vegetable Casserole

Prep time: 45 minutes | Cook time: 43 minutes |Serves 4

- 10 oz tofu, pressed and cubed
- 2 tsp olive oil
- 1 cup leeks, chopped
- 1 garlic clove, minced
- ½ cup celery, chopped
- ½ cup carrot, chopped
- 1 ½ pounds Brussels sprouts, shredded
- 1 habanero pepper, chopped
- 2 ½ cups mushrooms, sliced
- 1 ½ cups vegetable stock
- 2 tomatoes, chopped
- 2 thyme sprigs, chopped
- 1 rosemary sprig, chopped
- 2 bay leaves
- Salt and ground black pepper to taste

1. Set a pot over medium heat and warm oil. Add in garlic and leeks and sauté until soft and translucent, about 3 minutes. Add in tofu and cook for another 4 minutes. Add the habanero pepper, celery, mushrooms, and carrots.
2. Cook as you stir for 5 minutes. Stir in the rest of the ingredients. Simmer for 25 to 35 minutes or until cooked through. Remove and discard the bay leaves.

PER SERVING

Cal: 328 | Fat 18.5g | Net Carbs: 9.7g | Protein 21g

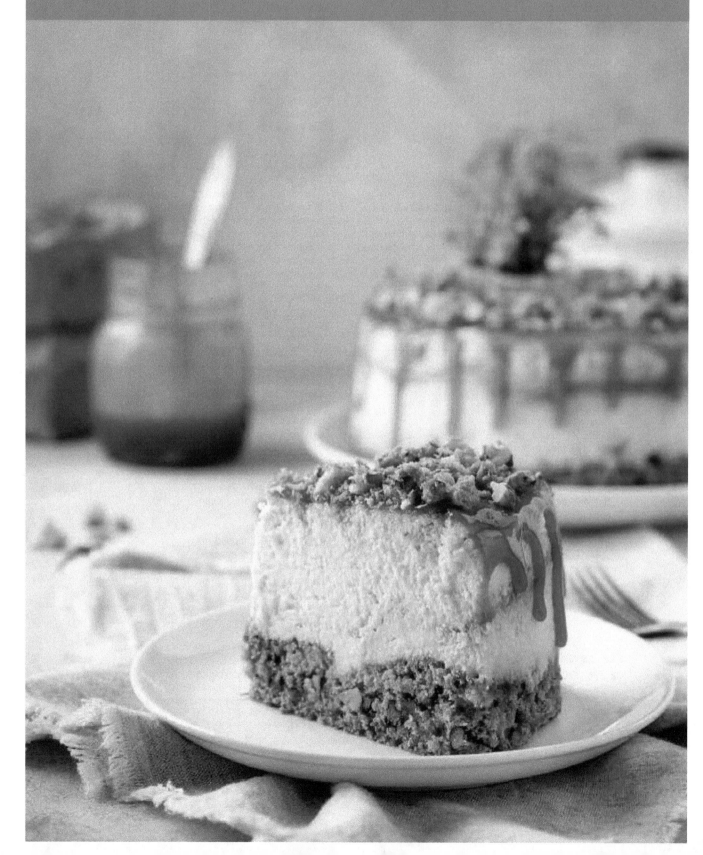

Chapter 10
Desserts

Coconut Panna Cotta with Cream & Caramel

Prep time: 10 minutes | Cook time: 5 minutes |Serves 4

- 4 eggs
- 1/3 cup erythritol, for caramel
- 2 cups coconut milk
- 1 tbsp vanilla extract
- 1 tbsp lemon zest
- ½ cup erythritol, for custard
- 2 cup heavy whipping cream
- Mint leaves, to serve

1. In a deep pan, heat the erythritol for the caramel. Add two tablespoons of water and bring to a boil. Lower the heat and cook until the caramel turns to a golden brown color.
2. Divide between 4 metal tins, set aside and let cool. In a bowl, mix the eggs, remaining erythritol, lemon zest, and vanilla. Beat in the coconut milk until well combined.
3. Pour the custard into each caramel-lined ramekin and place them into a deep baking tin.
4. Fill over the way with the remaining hot water. Bake at 350 F for around 45 minutes.
5. Take out the ramekins with tongs and refrigerate for at least 3 hours. Run a knife slowly around the edges to invert onto a dish. Serve with dollops of whipped cream and scattered with mint leaves.

PER SERVING

Cal: 268 | Fat: 31g | Net Carbs: 2.5g | Protein 6.5g

Superfood Red Smoothie

Prep time: 6 minutes | Cook time: 2 minutes |Serves 2

- 1 Granny Smith apple, chopped
- 1 cup strawberries
- 1 cup blueberries
- 2 small beets, peeled and chopped
- 2/3 cup ice cubes
- ½ lemon, juiced
- 2 cups almond milk

1. For the strawberries for garnishing, make a single deep cut on their sides, and set aside. In a smoothie maker, add the apples, strawberries, blueberries, beets, almond milk, and ice and blend the ingredients at high speed until nice and smooth, for about 75 seconds.
2. Add the lemon juice, and puree further for 30 seconds. Pour the drink into tall smoothie glasses, fix the reserved strawberries on each glass rim and serve with a straw.

PER SERVING

Cal: 233 | Fat: 4.3g | Net Carbs: 11.3g | Protein 5g

Vegan Chocolate Smoothie

Prep time: 10 minutes | Cook time: 5 minutes |Serves 2

- ¼ cup pumpkin seeds
- ¾ cup coconut milk
- ¼ cup water
- 1½ cups watercress
- 2 tsp vegan protein powder
- 1 tbsp chia seeds
- 1 tbsp unsweetened cocoa powder

1. In a blender, add all ingredients except for the chia seeds and process until creamy and uniform.
2. Place into two glasses, dust with chia seeds and chill before serving.

PER SERVING

Cal: 335 | Fat 29.7g Net Carbs 5.7g | Protein 6.5g

Power Green Smoothie

Prep time: 5 minutes | Cook time: 1 minutes |Serves 2

- 1 cup collard greens, chopped
- 3 stalks celery, chopped
- 1 ripe avocado, skinned, pitted, sliced
- 1 cup ice cubes
- 2 cups spinach, chopped
- 1 large cucumber, peeled and chopped
- Chia seeds to garnish

1. Add the collard greens, celery, avocado, and ice cubes in a blender, and blend for 50
2. seconds. Add the spinach and cucumber, and process for another 40 seconds until smooth.
3. Transfer the smoothie into glasses, garnish with chia seeds and serve right away.

PER SERVING

Cal: 187 | Fat: 12g | Net Carbs: 7.6g | Protein 3.2g

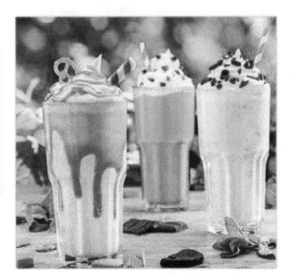

Chocolate Mousse with Cherries

Prep time: 45 minutes | Cook time: 26 minutes |Serves 4

- 8 eggs, separated into yolks and whites
- 12 oz unsweetened dark chocolate
- 2 tbsp salt
- ¾ cup swerve sugar
- ½ cup olive oil
- 3 tbsp brewed coffee
- Cherries
- 1 cup cherries, pitted and halved
- ½ stick cinnamon
- ½ cup water
- ½ lime, juiced

1. In a bowl, add the chocolate and melt in the microwave for 95 seconds. In a separate bowl, whisk the yolks with half of the swerve sugar until a pale yellow has formed, then, beat in the salt, olive oil, and coffee. Mix in the melted chocolate until smooth.
2. In a third bowl, whisk the whites with the hand mixer until a soft peak has formed. Sprinkle the remaining swerve sugar over and gently fold in with a spatula. Fetch a tablespoon of the chocolate mixture and fold in to combine. Pour in the remaining chocolate mixture and whisk to mix. Ladle the mousse into ramekins, cover with plastic wrap, and refrigerate overnight.
3. The next day, pour ½ cup of water, ½ cup of swerve, ½ stick cinnamon, and lime juice in a saucepan and bring to a simmer for 4 minutes, stirring to ensure the swerve has dissolved and a syrup has formed. Add cherries and poach in the sweetened water for 20 minutes until soft. Turn heat off and discard the cinnamon stick. Spoon a plum each with syrup on the chocolate mousse and serve.

PER SERVING

Cal: 288 | Fat: 23.4g | Net Carbs: 8.1g | Protein 10g

Strawberry Chocolate Mousse

Prep time: 30 minutes | Cook time: 30 minutes |Serves 4

- 6 eggs
- 1 cup dark chocolate chips
- 2 cups heavy cream
- 2 cups fresh strawberries, sliced
- 1 vanilla extract
- 1 tbsp xylitol

1. In a bowl, melt the chocolate in the microwave for a minute on high and let it cool for 10 minutes.
2. In another bowl, whip the cream until very soft. Add the eggs, vanilla extract, and xylitol; whisk to combine. Fold in the cooled chocolate. Divide the mousse between glasses, top with the strawberry slices and chill in the fridge for at least 30 minutes before serving.

PER SERVING

Cal: 567 | Fat: 45.6g | Net Carbs: 9.6g | Protein 13.6g

Minty Lemon Tart

Prep time: 50 minutes | Cook time: 40 minutes | Serves 4

- PieCrust
- ¼ cup almond flour
- 3 tbsp coconut flour
- ½ tsp salt
- ¼ cup butter, cold and crumbled
- 3 tbsp erythritol
- 1 ½ tsp vanilla extract
- 4 whole eggs
- Filling
- 4 tbsp melted butter
- 3 tsp swerve brown sugar
- 1 cup fresh blackberries
- 1 tsp vanilla extract
- 1 lemon, juiced
- 1 cup ricotta cheese
- 3 to 4 fresh mint leaves to garnish
- 1 egg, lightly beaten

1. In a large bowl, mix the almond flour, coconut flour, and salt.
2. Add the butter and mix with an electric hand mixer until crumbly. Add the erythritol and vanilla extract until mixed in. Then, pour in the 4 eggs one after another while mixing until formed into a ball. Flatten the dough a clean flat surface, cover in plastic wrap, and refrigerate for 1 hour.
3. Preheat the oven to 350 F and grease a pie pan with cooking spray. Lightly dust a clean flat surface with almond flour, unwrap the dough, and roll out the dough into a 1-inch diameter circle.
4. In a 10-inch shallow baking pan, mix the butter, swerve brown sugar, blackberries, vanilla extract, and lemon juice. Arrange the blackberries uniformly across the pan.
5. Lay the pastry over the fruit filling and tuck the sides into the pan. Brush with the beaten egg and bake in the oven for 35 to 40 minutes or until the golden and puffed up.
6. Remove, allow cooling for 5 minutes, and then run a knife around the pan to losing the pastry. Turn the pie over onto a plate, crumble the ricotta cheese on top, and garnish with the mint leaves.

PER SERVING

Cal: 533 | Fat 44g | Net Carbs 8.7g | Protein 17g

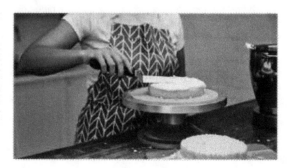

Almond Milk Berry Shake

Prep time: 5 minutes | Cook time: 5 minutes | Serves 2

- ½ cup fresh blueberries
- ½ cup raspberries
- ½ cup almond milk
- ¼ cup heavy cream
- Maple syrup to taste, sugar-free
- 1 tbsp sesame seeds
- Chopped pistachios for topping
- 1 tsp chopped mint leaves

1. Combine the blueberries, milk, heavy cream, and syrup in a blender. Process until smooth and pour into serving glasses. Top with the sesame seeds, pistachios, and mint leaves.
2. Serve immediately.

PER SERVING

Cal: 228g | Fat 21g | Net Carbs 5.4g | Protein 7.9g

No-Bake Raw Coconut Balls

Prep time: 22 minutes | Cook time: 20 minutes | Serves 4

- ¼ tsp coconut extract
- 2/3 cup melted coconut oil
- 15-oz can coconut milk
- 16 drops stevia liquid
- 1 cup unsweetened coconut flakes

1. In a bowl, mix the coconut oil with the milk, coconut extract, and stevia to combine. Stir in the coconut flakes until well distributed.
2. Pour into silicone muffin molds and freeze for 1 hour to harden.

PER SERVING

Cal: 211 | Fat: 19g | Net Carbs: 2.2g | Protein 2.9g

Quick Raspberry Vanilla Shake

Prep time: 2 minutes | Cook time: 2 minutes | Serves 2

- 2 cups raspberries
- 2 tbsp erythritol
- 6 raspberries to garnish
- ½ cup cold unsweetened almond milk
- 2/3 tsp vanilla extract
- ½ cup heavy whipping cream

1. In a large blender, process the raspberries, milk, vanilla extract, whipping cream, and erythritol for 2 minutes; work in two batches if needed.
2. The shake should be frosty. Pour into glasses, stick in straws, garnish with raspberries and serve.

PER SERVING

Cal: 213 | Fat: 13.4g | Net Carbs: 7.7g | Protein 4.5g

Almond Drunk Crumble

Prep time: 55 minutes | Cook time: 45 minutes | Serves 4

- 1 cup raspberries
- ½ teaspoon cinnamon
- ¼ cup erythritol, divided
- ½ tsp almond extract
- ½ cup red wine
- ½ cup salted butter, cubed
- 1 cup almond flour
- 2 tbsp ground almonds

1. In a baking dish, add raspberries, except for 5 for garnish, half of erythritol, almond extract, and stir.
2. In a bowl, rub the butter with the almond flour, and the remaining erythritol, and almonds until it resembles large breadcrumbs. Spoon the mixture to cover the raspberries, place in the oven, and bake in the oven for 45 minutes at 375 F until the top looks golden brown.
3. Remove, let cool for 3 minutes, and serve topped with the reserved raspberries.

PER SERVING

Cal: 213 | Fat 16.4g | Net Carbs 8.5g | Protein 1.3g :

Peanut Butter Ice Cream

Prep time: 50 minutes | Cook time: 50 minutes | Serves 4

- ½ cup smooth peanut butter
- ½ cup erythritol
- 3 cups half and half
- 1 tsp vanilla extract
- 1 pinch of salt
- ½ cups raspberries

1. In a bowl, beat peanut butter and erythritol with a hand mixer until smooth. Gradually whisk in half and half until thoroughly combined. Add in vanilla and salt and mix.
2. Transfer the mixture to a loaf pan and freeze for 50 minutes until firmed up. Scoop into glasses when ready and serve topped with raspberries.

PER SERVING

Cal: 436 | Fat: 38.5g | Net Carbs: 9.5g | Protein 13g

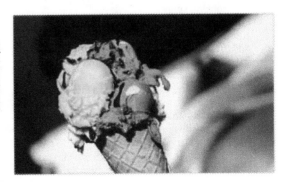

Refreshing Strawberry Lemonade with Basil

Prep time: 3 minutes | Cook time: 1 minutes | Serves 4

- 2 cups water
- 12 strawberries, leaves removed
- ¼ cup fresh lemon juice
- 1/3 cup fresh mint, reserve some for garnishing
- ½ cup erythritol
- Crushed Ice
- Halved strawberries to garnish
- Basil leaves to garnish

1. Add some ice into 2 serving glasses and set aside. In a pitcher of a blender, add water, strawberries, lemon juice, mint, and erythritol. Process the ingredients for 30 seconds. The mixture should be pink and the mint finely chopped. Adjust the taste and divide between the ice glasses.
2. Drop 2 strawberry halves and basil leaves in each glass and serve immediately.

PER SERVING

Cal: 36 | Fat: 0.7g | Net Carbs: 5.1g | Protein 1.5g

Quick Vanilla Tart

Prep time: 75 minutes | Cook time: 50 minutes | Serves 4

- Pie Crust
- ¼ cup almond flour + extra for dusting
- 3 tbsp coconut flour
- ½ tsp salt
- ¼ cup butter, cold and crumbled
- 3 tbsp erythritol
- 1½ tsp vanilla extract
- 4 whole eggs
- Filling
- 2 whole eggs + 3 egg yolks
- ½ cup swerve sugar
- 1 tsp vanilla bean paste
- 2 tbsp coconut flour
- 1¼ cup almond milk
- 1¼ cup heavy cream
- 1½ tbsp maple syrup, sugar-free
- ¼ cup chopped almonds

1. Preheat the oven to 350 F and grease a pie pan with cooking spray.
2. In a large bowl, mix the almond flour, coconut flour, and salt.
3. Add the butter and mix with an electric hand mixer until crumbly. Add the erythritol and vanilla extract until mixed in. Then, pour in the 4 eggs one after another while mixing until formed into a ball.
4. Flatten the dough a clean flat surface, cover in plastic wrap, and refrigerate for 1 hour.
5. After, lightly dust a clean flat surface with almond flour, unwrap the dough, and roll out the dough into a large rectangle, ½ - inch thickness and fit into a pie pan. Bake in the oven until golden.

Remove after and allow cooling.

6. In a large mixing bowl, whisk the whole 3 eggs, egg yolks, swerve sugar, vanilla bean paste, and coconut flour. Put the almond milk, heavy cream, and maple syrup into a medium pot and bring to a boil over medium heat. Pour the mixture into the egg mixture and whisk while pouring.
7. Run the batter through a fine strainer into a bowl and skim off any froth.
8. Take out the pie pastry from the oven, pour out the baking beans, remove the parchment paper, and transfer the egg batter into the pie. Bake in the oven for 40 to 50 minutes or until the custard sets with a slight wobble in the center. Garnish with the chopped almonds, slice, and serve when cooled.

PER SERVING

Cal: 542 | Fat 41g | Net Carbs 8.5g | Protein 16g

Cranberry Granola Bars

Prep time: 50 minutes | Cook time: 45 minutes | Serves 4

- 1 cup hazelnuts and walnuts, chopped
- 2 tbsp dried cranberries
- ¼ cup flax meal
- ¼ cup coconut milk
- ¼ cup poppy seeds
- ¼ cup pumpkin seeds
- 4 drops stevia
- ¼ cup coconut oil, melted
- ½ tsp vanilla paste
- ½ tsp ground cloves
- ½ tsp grated nutmeg
- ½ tsp lemon zest

1. Preheat oven to 280 F and line a baking sheet with parchment paper. In a large mixing bowl, combine all ingredients with ¼ cup of water and stir to coat. Spread the mixture onto the baking sheet.
2. Bake for 45 minutes, stirring at intervals of 15 minutes. Let cool at room temperature. Cut into bars to serve.

PER SERVING

Cal: 451 | Fat 43g | Net Carbs: 6.3g | Protein 10.2g

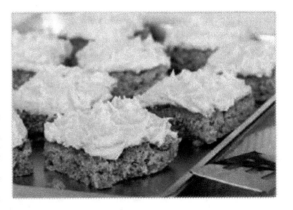

Hazelnut & Chocolate Cake

Prep time: 10 minutes | Cook time: 45 minutes | Serves 4

- ½ cup olive oil
- 1 cup almond flour
- ½ cup unsweetened dark chocolate, melted
- 2 tsp hazelnut extract
- 2 tsp cinnamon powder
- ½ cup boiling water
- 3 large eggs
- ¼ cup ground hazelnuts
- 1 tbsp unsweetened dark chocolate, shaved

1. Preheat oven to 350 F and grease a baking pan with cooking spray and line with parchment paper. In a large bowl, combine the olive oil, almond flour, chocolate, swerve sugar, hazelnut extract, salt, cinnamon powder, and boiling water. Crack the eggs one after the other while beating until smooth.
2. Pour the batter into the springform pan and bake in the oven for 45 minutes or until a toothpick inserted comes out clean. Take out from the oven; allow cooling in the pan for 10 minutes, then turn over onto a wire rack. Sprinkle with ground hazelnuts and shaved chocolate, slice, and serve.

PER SERVING

Cal: 505 | Fat 46.5g | Net Carbs 8g | Protein 6.1g

Grandma's Zucchini & Nut Cake

Prep time: 30 minutes | Cook time: 40 minutes | Serves 4

- 1 cup butter, softened + extra for greasing
- 1 cup erythritol
- 4 eggs
- 2/3 cup coconut flour
- 2 tsp baking powder
- 2/3 cup ground almonds
- 1 lemon, zested and juiced
- 1 cup crème fraiche, for serving
- 1 tbsp chopped walnuts

1. Grease a springform pan with cooking spray, and line with parchment paper.
2. In a bowl, beat the butter and erythritol until creamy and pale. Add the eggs one after another while whisking. Sift the coconut flour and baking powder into the mixture and stir along with the ground almonds, lemon zest, juice, and zucchini.
3. Preheat oven to 375 F. Spoon the mixture into the springform pan and bake in the oven for 40 minutes or until risen and a toothpick inserted into the cake comes out clean.
4. Remove the cake from the oven when ready; allow cooling for 10 minutes, and transfer to a wire rack. Spread the crème fraiche on top of the cake and sprinkle with the walnuts. Slice and serve.

PER SERVING

Cal: 778 | Fat 65g | Net Carbs 9g | Protein 29.2g

Sage Chocolate Cheese Cake

Prep time: 15 minutes | Cook time: 14 minutes | Serves 4

CRUST

- 1 cup raw almonds
- ½ cup salted butter, melted
- 2 tbsp swerve sugar

CAKE

- 4 tbsp unsalted butter, melted
- 2 gelatine sheets
- 2 tbsp lime juice
- 2/3 cup unsweetened dark chocolate, chopped
- 2 tbsp cocoa powder
- 1 ½ cups cream cheese
- ½ cup swerve sugar
- 1 cup Greek yogurt
- 1 fresh sage leaf, chopped

1. Preheat oven to 350 F.
2. In a blender, process the almonds until finely ground. Add the butter and sweetener, and mix until combined. Press the crust mixture into the bottom of the cake pan until firm. Bake for 5 minutes. Place in the fridge to chill afterward.
3. In a small pot, combine the gelatin with the lime juice, and a tablespoon of water. Allow sitting for 5 minutes and then, place the pot over medium heat to dissolve the gelatin. Set aside.
4. Pour the dark chocolate in a bowl and melt in the microwave for 1 minute, stirring at every 10 seconds interval. Set aside.
5. In another, beat the cream cheese and swerve sugar using an electric mixer until smooth.
6. Stir in the yogurt and gelatin until evenly combined. Fold in the melted dark chocolate and then the sage leaf.
7. Remove the pan from the fridge and pour the cream mixture on top. Tap the side gently to release any trapped air bubbles and transfer to the fridge to chip for 3 hours or more. Dust the cake with cocoa powder and slice to serve.

PER SERVING

Cal: 675 | Fat 53g | Net Carbs 13g | Protein 21g

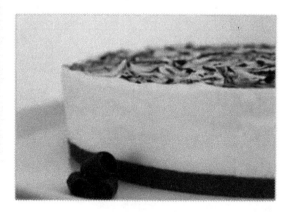

Appendix 1 Measurement Conversion Chart

Volume Equivalents (Dry)	
US STANDARD	**METRIC (APPROXIMATE)**
1/8 teaspoon	0.5 mL
1/4 teaspoon	1 mL
1/2 teaspoon	2 mL
3/4 teaspoon	4 mL
1 teaspoon	5 mL
1 tablespoon	15 mL
1/4 cup	59 mL
1/2 cup	118 mL
3/4 cup	177 mL
1 cup	235 mL
2 cups	475 mL
3 cups	700 mL
4 cups	1 L

Volume Equivalents (Liquid)		
US STANDARD	**US STANDARD (OUNCES)**	**METRIC (APPROXIMATE)**
2 tablespoons	1 fl.oz.	30 mL
1/4 cup	2 fl.oz.	60 mL
1/2 cup	4 fl.oz.	120 mL
1 cup	8 fl.oz.	240 mL
1 1/2 cup	12 fl.oz.	355 mL
2 cups or 1 pint	16 fl.oz.	475 mL
4 cups or 1 quart	32 fl.oz.	1 L
1 gallon	128 fl.oz.	4 L

Temperatures Equivalents	
FAHRENHEIT(F)	**CELSIUS(C) APPROXIMATE)**
225 °F	107 °C
250 °F	120 ° °C
275 °F	135 °C
300 °F	150 °C
325 °F	160 °C
350 °F	180 °C
375 °F	190 °C
400 °F	205 °C
425 °F	220 °C
450 °F	235 °C
475 °F	245 °C
500 °F	260 °C

Weight Equivalents	
US STANDARD	**METRIC (APPROXIMATE)**
1 ounce	28 g
2 ounces	57 g
5 ounces	142 g
10 ounces	284 g
15 ounces	425 g
16 ounces (1 pound)	455 g
1.5 pounds	680 g
2 pounds	907 g

Appendix 2 The Dirty Dozen and Clean Fifteen

The Environmental Working Group (EWG) is a nonprofit, nonpartisan organization dedicated to protecting human health and the environment Its mission is to empower people to live healthier lives in a healthier environment. This organization publishes an annual list of the twelve kinds of produce, in sequence, that have the highest amount of pesticide residue-the Dirty Dozen-as well as a list of the fifteen kinds ofproduce that have the least amount of pesticide residue-the Clean Fifteen.

THE DIRTY DOZEN	
The 2016 Dirty Dozen includes the following produce. These are considered among the year's most important produce to buy organic:	
Strawberries	Spinach
Apples	Tomatoes
Nectarines	Bell peppers
Peaches	Cherry tomatoes
Celery	Cucumbers
Grapes	Kale/collard greens
Cherries	Hot peppers
The Dirty Dozen list contains two additional itemskale/collard greens and hot peppers-because they tend to contain trace levels of highly hazardous pesticides.	

THE CLEAN FIFTEEN	
The least critical to buy organically are the Clean Fifteen list. The following are on the 2016 list:	
Avocados	Papayas
Corn	Kiw
Pineapples	Eggplant
Cabbage	Honeydew
Sweet peas	Grapefruit
Onions	Cantaloupe
Asparagus	Cauliflower
Mangos	
Some of the sweet corn sold in the United States are made from genetically engineered (GE) seedstock. Buy organic varieties of these crops to avoid GE produce.	

Appendix 3 Index

A

all-purpose flour 50, 53
allspice 15
almond 5, 14
ancho chile 10
ancho chile powder 5
apple 9
apple cider vinegar 9
arugula 51
avocado 11

B

bacon 52
balsamic vinegar 7, 12, 52
basil 5, 8, 11, 13
beet 52
bell pepper 50, 51, 53
black beans 50, 51
broccoli 51, 52, 53
buns 52
butter 50

C

canola oil 50, 51, 52
carrot 52, 53
cauliflower 5, 52
cayenne 5, 52
cayenne pepper 52
Cheddar cheese 52
chicken 6
chili powder 50, 51
chipanle pepper 50
chives 5, 6, 52
cinnamon 15
coconut 6
Colby Jack cheese 51
coriander 52
corn 50, 51
corn kernels 50
cumin 5, 10, 15, 50, 51, 52

D

diced panatoes 50
Dijon mustard 7, 12, 13, 51
dry onion powder 52

E

egg 14, 50, 53
enchilada sauce 51

F

fennel seed 53
flour 50, 53
fresh chives 5, 6, 52
fresh cilantro 52
fresh cilantro leaves 52
fresh dill 5
fresh parsley 6, 52
fresh parsley leaves 52

G

garlic 5, 9, 10, 11, 13, 14, 50, 51, 52, 53
garlic powder 8, 9, 52, 53

H

half-and-half 50
hemp seeds 8
honey 9, 51

I

instant rice 51

K

kale 14
kale leaves 14
ketchup 53
kosher salt 5, 10, 15

L

lemon 5, 6, 14, 51, 53
lemon juice 6, 8, 11, 13, 14, 51
lime 9, 12
lime juice 9, 12
lime zest 9, 12

M

maple syrup 7, 12, 53
Marinara Sauce 5
micro greens 52
milk 5, 50
mixed berries 12
Mozzarella 50, 53
Mozzarella cheese 50, 53
mushroom 51, 52
mustard 51, 53
mustard powder 53

N

nutritional yeast 5

O

olive oil 5, 12, 13, 14, 50, 51, 52, 53
onion 5, 50, 51
onion powder 8
oregano 5, 8, 10, 50

P

panatoes 50, 52
paprika 5, 15, 52
Parmesan cheese 51, 53
parsley 6, 52
pesto 52
pink Himalayan salt 5, 7, 8, 11
pizza dough 50, 53
pizza sauce 50
plain coconut yogurt 6
plain Greek yogurt 5
porcini powder 53
potato 53

R

Ranch dressing 52
raw honey 9, 12, 13
red pepper flakes 5, 8, 14, 15, 51, 53
ricotta cheese 53

S

saffron 52
Serrano pepper 53
sugar 10
summer squash 51

T

tahini 5, 8, 9, 11
thyme 50
toasted almonds 14
tomato 5, 50, 52, 53
turmeric 15

U

unsalted butter 50
unsweetened almond milk 5

V

vegetable broth 50
vegetable stock 51

W

white wine 8, 11
wine vinegar 8, 10, 11

Y

yogurt 5, 6

Z

zucchini 50, 51, 52, 53

BROOKE B. ORDUNA